WHO/NHD/01.08
WHO/FCH/CAH/01.23
ORIGINAL: ENGLISH
DISTR.: GENERAL

THE OPTIMAL DURATION OF EXCLUSIVE BREASTFEEDING
A SYSTEMATIC REVIEW

MICHAEL S. KRAMER, MD
RITSUKO KAKUMA, MSc

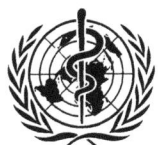

DEPARTMENT OF NUTRITION FOR HEALTH AND DEVELOPMENT
DEPARTMENT OF CHILD AND ADOLESCENT HEALTH AND DEVELOPMENT
WORLD HEALTH ORGANIZATION

© World Health Organization, 2002

This document is not a formal publication of the World Health Organization (WHO), and all rights are reserved by the Organization. The document may, however, be freely reviewed, abstracted, reproduced and translated, in part or in whole, but not for sale for use in conjunction with commercial purposes.

The views expressed in documents by named authors are solely the responsibility of those authors.

Designed by minimum graphics
Printed in Switzerland

Contents

Abstract	1
Introduction	3
Search methods	5
Selection criteria for studies	5
Types of intervention/exposure	5
Types of outcome measures	5
Search strategy for identification of studies	5
Selection of studies for inclusion	6
Review methods	9
Description of studies	9
Methodologic quality of included studies	9
Data collection	10
Data analysis	10
Results	14
Comparison 1: Controlled trials of exclusive vs mixed breastfeeding for 4–6 months, developing countries	14
Comparison 2: Observational studies of exclusive vs mixed breastfeeding for 3–7 months, developing countries	15
Comparison 3: Observational studies of exclusive vs mixed breastfeeding for 3–7 months, developed countries	16
Discussion	19
Summary of findings	19
Implications for future research	19
Conclusion	19
References	21
Annexes	25
Annex 1. Comparison 01: Exclusive vs mixed breastfeeding 4–6 months, developing countries, controlled trials	25
Annex 2. Comparison 02: Exclusive vs mixed breastfeeding 3–7 months, developing countries, observational studies	32
Annex 3. Comparison 03: Exclusive vs mixed breastfeeding 3–7 months, developed countries, observational studies	36

Abstract

Background: The longstanding debate over the optimal duration of exclusive breastfeeding has centered on the so-called "weanling's dilemma" in developing countries: the choice between the known protective effect of exclusive breastfeeding against infectious morbidity and the (theoretical) insufficiency of breast milk alone to satisfy the infant's energy and micronutrient requirements beyond 4 months of age. The debate over whether to recommend exclusive breastfeeding for 4–6 months vs "about 6 months" has recently become more intense.

Objectives: The primary objective of this review was to assess the effects on child health, growth, and development, and on maternal health, of exclusive breastfeeding for 6 months vs exclusive breastfeeding for 3–4 months with mixed breastfeeding (introduction of complementary liquid or solid foods with continued breastfeeding) thereafter through 6 months.

Search strategy: Two independent literature searches were carried out, together comprising the following databases: MEDLINE (as of 1966), Index Medicus (prior to 1966), CINAHL, HealthSTAR, BIOSIS, CAB Abstracts, EMBASE-Medicine, EMBASE-Psychology, Econlit, Index Medicus for the WHO Eastern Mediterranean Region, African Index Medicus, Lilacs (Latin American and Carribean literature), EBM Reviews-Best Evidence, the Cochrane Database of Systematic Reviews, and the Cochrane Controlled Trials Register. No language restrictions were imposed. The two searches yielded a total of 2,668 unique citations. Contacts with experts in the field yielded additional published and unpublished studies.

Selection criteria: We selected all internally-controlled clinical trials and observational studies comparing child or maternal health outcomes with exclusive breastfeeding for 6 or more months vs exclusive breastfeeding for at least 3–4 months with continued mixed breastfeeding until at least 6 months. Studies were stratified according to study design (controlled trials vs observational studies), provenance (developing vs developed countries), and timing of compared feeding groups (3–7 months vs later).

Data collection and analysis: Two reviewers independently assessed study quality (using *a priori* assessment criteria) and extracted data.

Main results: Sixteen independent studies meeting the selection criteria were identified by the literature search: 7 from developing countries (2 of which were controlled trials in Honduras) and 9 from developed countries (all observational studies). The two trials did not receive high methodologic quality ratings but were nonetheless superior to any of the observational studies included in this review. The observational studies were of variable quality; in addition, their nonexperimental designs were not able to exclude potential sources of confounding and selection bias. Definitions of exclusive breastfeeding varied considerably across studies. Neither the trials nor the observational studies suggest that infants who continue to be exclusively breastfed for 6 months show deficits in weight or length gain, although larger sample sizes would be required to rule out small increases in the risk of undernutrition. The data are scarce with respect to iron status, but at least in developing country settings where newborn iron stores may be suboptimal, suggest that exclusive breastfeeding without iron supplementation through 6 months may compromise hematologic status. Based primarily on an observational analysis of a large randomized trial in Belarus, infants who continue exclusive breastfeeding for 6 months or more appear to have a significantly reduced risk of one or more episodes of gastrointestinal infection. No significant reduction in risk of atopic eczema, asthma, or other atopic outcomes has been demonstrated in studies from Finland, Australia, and Belarus. Data from the two Honduran trials suggest that exclusive breastfeeding through 6 months is associated with delayed resumption of menses and more rapid postpartum weight loss in the mother.

Reviewers' conclusions: We found no objective evidence of a "weanling's dilemma." Infants who are exclusively breastfed for 6 months experience less morbidity from gastrointestinal infection than those who are mixed breastfed as of 3 or 4 months, and no deficits have been demonstrated in growth among infants from either developing or developed countries who are exclusively breastfed for 6 months. Moreover, the mothers of such infants have more prolonged lactational amenorrhea. Although infants should still be managed individually so that insufficient growth or other adverse outcomes are not ignored and appropriate interventions are provided, the available evidence demonstrates no apparent risks in recommending, as public health policy, exclusive breastfeeding for the first 6 months of life in both developing and developed country settings. Large randomized trials are recommended in both types of setting to rule out small adverse effects on growth and to confirm the reported health benefits of exclusive breastfeeding for 6 months.

Introduction

The debate over the optimal duration of exclusive breastfeeding has had a long history. Growth faltering is a commonly observed phenomenon in developing countries after about 3 months of age.[1,2] This growth faltering has traditionally been attributed to three factors: (1) the inadequacy of energy intake from breast milk alone after 3 or 4 months; (2) the poor nutritional quality (i.e., low energy and micronutrient content) of the complementary foods commonly introduced in many developing countries; and (3) the adverse effects of infection on energy intake and expenditure. The inadequacy of breast milk for energy requirements beyond 3 or 4 months was initially based on calculations made by the Food and Agricultural Organization (FAO) and World Health Organization (WHO) in 1973.[3] More careful studies since the 1980s[4-7] and a later FAO/WHO report,[8] however, have shown that the earlier FAO/WHO figures substantially overestimate true energy requirements in infancy.[4-7]

The belief that breast milk alone is nutritionally insufficient after 3 or 4 months, combined with the fact that complementary foods given in many developing countries are both nutritionally inadequate and contaminated, led to concern about the so-called "weanling's dilemma."[9,10] Breastfeeding is a life-and-death issue in developing countries. A recent meta-analysis[11] reported markedly reduced mortality (especially due to infectious disease) with breastfeeding even into the second year of life. A recent study from India reported an increased risk of postneonatal mortality associated with exclusive breastfeeding >3 months,[12] but reverse causality (illness prior to death preventing the infant's acceptance of complementary foods), selection bias (exclusion of infants who died prior to each cross-sectional period), or uncontrolled confounding might explain this result.

The weanling's dilemma and the risk of mortality associated with early introduction of complementary foods are concerns primarily in developing countries. In most developed countries, uncontaminated, nutritionally adequate complementary foods are readily available, and growth faltering is relatively uncommon. With the resurgence of breastfeeding in developed countries, however, recent attention has turned to the importance of promoting its duration and exclusivity.

The epidemiologic evidence is now overwhelming that, even in developed countries, breastfeeding protects against gastrointestinal and (to a lesser extent) respiratory infection, and that the protective effect is enhanced with greater duration and exclusivity of breastfeeding.[13-17] ("Greater duration and exclusivity" is used in a general sense here; the references cited do not pertain specifically to the subject of this review, i.e., the optimal duration of exclusive breastfeeding.) Prolonged and exclusive breastfeeding has also been associated with a reduced risk of the sudden infant death syndrome (SIDS)[18] and of atopic disease,[19-21] and some studies even suggest acceleration of neurocognitive development[22-28] and protection against long-term chronic conditions and diseases like obesity,[29-31] type I diabetes mellitus,[32,33] Crohn's disease,[34] and lymphoma.[35,36] Maternal health benefits have also received considerable attention in developed countries, including possible protection against breast cancer among premenopausal women,[37-39] ovarian cancer,[40] and osteoporosis.[41-43]

Although growth faltering is uncommon in developed countries, a recent pooled analysis of U.S., Canadian, and European data sets undertaken by the WHO Working Group on Infant Growth showed that infants from developed countries who follow current WHO feeding recommendations (to exclusively breastfeed for 4 to 6 months of age and to continue breastfeeding with adequate complementary foods up to 2 years of age) show a deceleration in both weight and length gain relative to the international WHO/NCHS growth reference from around 3 to 12 months, with partial catch-up in the second year.[44,45] More recent studies, including a Danish population-based cohort study,[46] an analysis based on the third U.S. National Health and Nutrition Examination Survey,[47] and the Euro-Growth study[48] have also reported an association between prolonged and exclusive breastfeeding and slower growth during infancy. Unfortunately, the current WHO/NCHS reference is based on the Fels Longitudinal Study, which was conducted many decades ago in infants who were primarily bottle-fed. WHO has therefore embarked on an ambitious study to establish new growth standards for infants following current feeding recommendations.[49,50] In developed country settings, it is not at all clear that the more rapid growth reported in infants who are formula-fed, or breastfed less exclusively and for a shorter duration, is an advantage. Moreover, a recent, large randomized trial from Belarus has reported that breastfed infants born and followed at sites randomized to a breastfeeding promotion intervention (and who were breastfed more exclusively and for a longer duration) actually grew more rapidly in the first 6–9 months than those born and followed at control (nonintervention) sites.[51,52,53]

In the last years, recommendations for the optimal duration of exclusive breastfeeding promoted by WHO and UNICEF started to differ. WHO had continued to recommend exclusive breastfeeding for 4 to 6 months, with the introduction of complementary foods thereafter,[54] whereas UNICEF preferred the wording "for about 6 months."[55] This led to concerns in the larger infant nutrition and public health communities.[56] The American Academy of Pediatrics' position is unclear; in two different sections of their Pediatric Nutrition Handbook,[57] they alternatively recommend human milk "as the exclusive nutrient source ... during the first 6 months" (p. 18) and "to delay introduction of solid foods until 4 to 6 months" (p. 38).

Until recently, the only scientific evidence contributing to this debate was based on observational studies, with well-recognized sources of potential bias. Some of these biases tend to favor exclusively breastfed infants, while others favor those who receive earlier complementary feeding. Infants who continue to be exclusively breastfed tend to be those who remain healthy and on an acceptable growth trajectory; significant illness or growth faltering can lead to interruption of breastfeeding or supplementation with infant formula or solid foods.[58,59] Confounding by indication[60] [i.e., the **reason** (indication) for the supplementation affects the outcome, rather than the supplementation itself] is another important bias, and could operate in either direction. Poorly-growing infants (especially those in developing countries) are likely to receive complementary feedings earlier because of their slower growth. In developed countries, however, rapidly-growing infants may require more energy than can be met by the increasingly spaced feedings typical of such settings. This may result in crying and poor sleeping, supplementation with formula and/or solid foods, reduced suckling, and a vicious cycle leading to earlier termination of breastfeeding. Reverse causality is another potential source of bias, particularly with respect to infectious morbidity and neuromotor development.[61] Infants who develop a clinically important infection are likely to become anorectic and to reduce their breast milk intake, which can in turn lead to reduction in milk production and even termination of breastfeeding. This is particularly a problem in cross-sectional studies, because the temporal sequence of the early signs of infection and termination of breastfeeding may not be adequately appreciated; infection may be blamed on the termination of breastfeeding, rather than the reverse. Advanced neuromotor development may also lead to earlier induction of solid foods, which could then receive "credit" for accelerating motor development.[62] Finally, other unmeasured or poorly measured confounding variables could also bias the association between introduction of complementary foods and infant health outcomes.

Because of these well-recognized problems in observational studies, two recent controlled clinical trials[63,64] from Honduras have attracted considerable interest. These trials allocated infants born to either continue breastfeeding exclusively for 6 months or to receive solid foods along with continued breastfeeding from 4 months onwards. The results showed no significant benefit for growth nor any disadvantage for morbidity with the earlier introduction of complementary foods, but the small sample sizes and published analyses based on compliance with allocation (i.e., not on intention-to-treat) have prevented universal acceptance of these results.[65] In addition, the complementary foods used were those commonly found in developed countries, rather than in those traditionally used in Honduras or other developing countries.

Most studies have reported effects in terms of group differences in mean z-scores or in mean weight or length gain; few have provided data on the tails (extremes) of the distribution, e.g., anthropometric indices (z-scores <-2) of underweight, stunting, or wasting, and none (even the larger observational studies) has had a sufficient sample size to detect modest effects on these indices. In fact, there has been an underlying assumption in this field that "one size fits all," i.e., that average population effects can be applied to individual infants and that one international recommendation is therefore adequate for all infants. There has been little discussion of the fact that all infants, regardless of how they are fed, require careful monitoring of growth and illness, with appropriate interventions undertaken whenever clinically indicated. Because of the ongoing controversy and polarization over this issue, the World Health Organization requested, in the spring of 2000, a systematic review of the available evidence before considering a revision or continuation of its current infant feeding recommendations. In the remainder of this report, we summarize the methods, results, and conclusions of that review.

Search methods

Selection criteria for studies

We selected controlled clinical trials and observational studies, published in all languages, examining whether or not exclusive breastfeeding (EBF) until 6 months of age has an impact on growth, development, morbidity, and survival of healthy, term infants and their mothers. Studies of (or including) low-birth-weight (<2500 g) infants were not excluded, provided that such infants were born at term (≥37 completed weeks). Only those studies with an internal comparison group were included in the review, i.e., we excluded studies based on external comparisons (with reference data). The comparisons must have been based on one group of infants who received EBF for ≥3 but <7 months and mixed breastfeeding (MBF) until 6 months or later (i.e., infants were introduced to liquid or solid foods between 3 and 6 months of age), and another group of subjects who were exclusively breastfed for ≥6 months. This restriction was imposed to provide direct relevance to the clinical and public health decision context: whether infants who are exclusively breastfed for the first 3–4 months should continue EBF or should receive complementary foods in addition to breast milk (MBF). Thus studies comparing EBF and MBF from birth were excluded, as were those that investigated the effects of age at introduction of nonbreast milk liquid or solid foods but did not ensure EBF ≥3 months prior to their introduction.

Types of intervention/exposure

Among infants EBF for at least 3 months, the interventions/exposures compared were continued EBF vs MBF. The "complementary" foods used in MBF included juices, formula, other milks, other liquids, or solid foods. Although WHO defines EBF as breastfeeding with no supplemental liquids or solid foods other than medications or vitamins,[66] few studies strictly adhered to the WHO definition. In some studies, so-called "EBF" included provision of water, teas, or juices (corresponding to WHO's definition of predominant breastfeeding[66]) or even small amounts of infant formula. The definitions of EBF and MBF used in each study are described in the Table of Included Studies.

Types of outcome measures

No infant or maternal health outcomes were excluded from consideration. The infant outcomes specifically sought (but not necessarily found) included growth [weight, length, and head circumference and z-scores (based on the WHO/NCHS reference) for weight-for-age (WAZ), length-for-age (LAZ), and weight-for-length (WLZ)], infections, morbidity, mortality, micronutrient status, neuromotor and cognitive development, asthma, atopic eczema, other allergic diseases, Type 1 diabetes, blood pressure, and subsequent adult chronic diseases such as coronary heart disease, hypertension, Type 2 diabetes, and inflammatory and autoimmune diseases. Maternal outcomes sought included postpartum weight loss, duration of lactational amenorrhea, and such chronic diseases as breast and ovarian cancer and osteoporosis.

Search strategy for identification of studies

In order to capture as many relevant studies as possible, two independent literature searches were conducted: one by staff at the Department of Nutrition of WHO and one by the authors. The search details are shown below.

The search by WHO was conducted between June and August 2000 in the following databases: MEDLINE (1966 to June 2000), Pre-MEDLINE (Index Medicus previous to 1966), CINAHL (1982 to June 2000), HealthSTAR (1975 to August 2000), EBM Reviews-Best Evidence (1991 to July/August 2000), SocioFile (1974 to July 2000), Cochrane Database of Systematic Reviews (Issue 2, 2000), CAB Abstracts (1973 to July 2000), EMBASE-Psychology (1987 to 3rd Quarter, 2000), Econlit (1969 to August 2000), Index Medicus for the WHO Eastern Mediterranean (IMEMR), African Index Medicus (AIM), and Lilacs (Latin American and Caribbean literature).

Where applicable, the medical subject heading (MeSH) "breast feeding," and otherwise the free language terms "breast-feeding," "breast feeding," or "breastfeeding" combined with "exclusive" or "exclusively" were used in the search strategy. The search yielded 1,423 citations (MEDLINE 686, Pre-MEDLINE 15, CINAHL 25, HealthSTAR 1, EBM-Best Evidence 7, Socio File 2, Cochrane Database of Systematic Reviews 8, CAB Abstracts 680, EMBASE-Psychology 4, other databases 0). Once duplicates were removed, 1,035 citations remained; these were then assessed for eligibility.

The authors' search was conducted on August 12, 2000 in the following databases: MEDLINE (1966 to June 2000), CINAHL (1982 to April 2000), HealthSTAR (1975 to August 2000), BIOSIS (1989 to 2000), CAB Abstracts (1973 to June 2000), Cochrane Database of Systematic Reviews (Issue 3, 2000), Cochrane Controlled Trials Register (Issue 3, 2000), and EMBASE-Medicine (1980 to present).

The terms "breast feeding," "infant," and "growth," as MeSH headings and text words, were combined in the search strategy. This search yielded a total of 2,496 citations (MEDLINE yielded 1,079 citations, CINAHL 75, HealthSTAR 2, BIOSIS 190, CAB 614, Cochrane Database of Systematic Reviews 25, Cochrane Controlled Trials Register 122, and EMBASE 389). Once duplicates among the databases were removed, 1,845 citations remained, 1,633 of which were different from the 1,035 identified by the WHO search. Thus 2,668 unique citations were identified by the two searches.

For both searches, every effort was made to identify relevant non-English language articles and abstracts. Given their own backgrounds, the reviewers themselves were able to determine the eligibility of articles in French, Spanish, and Japanese. For publications in other languages, two options were available. Many articles in languages other than English provided English abstracts. As such, all potentially relevant articles were obtained and checked for availability of English abstracts. If such abstracts were not available, or were available but did not provide enough information to determine their eligibility, then assistance was requested from WHO to determine their eligibility for inclusion. No article or abstract was excluded because of language of publication.

In addition to the studies found through the two electronic searches, reference lists of identified articles were checked, and contacts with experts in the field were made to identify other potentially relevant published or unpublished studies. Attempts were made to contact the authors of all studies that qualified for inclusion in the review to obtain methodologic details, clarify inconsistencies, and obtain unpublished data.

Selection of studies for inclusion

Many studies were identified that either compared outcomes in infants receiving EBF vs MBF or investigated the effects of age at introduction of nonbreast-milk liquid or solid foods. The vast majority of these studies were ineligible for inclusion, however, because they did not ensure EBF ≥3 months prior to introducing these complementary foods in the MBF group and/or a comparison group with EBF ≥6 months.

We identified 32 unique citations (articles or abstracts) that met the selection criteria, comprising 16 separate studies. Of the 16 included studies, 7 were carried out in developing countries and the other 9 in developed countries.

Eight of the 32 total citations were found by both searches[63,64,67-72]; 7 were identified only by the WHO search[21,73-78]; 6 were found only by the authors' search.[45,62,79-82] Eleven additional citations were located through contacts with experts and reference lists of relevant articles.[7,44,51,53,83-88] The selected studies are listed below. They are generally referred to by the last name of the first author of the earliest citation for each study, along with the year of publication of that citation. Thirty-five references are listed; one[85] of the 32 unique citations appears twice, and another[7] 3 times.

Developing countries

Adair 1993

a. Adair L, Popkin BM, Vanderslice J, Akin J, Guilkey D, Black R, et al. Growth dynamics during the first two years of life: a prospective study in the Philippines. *Eur J Clin Nutr* 1993;47:42–51.[79]

b. Brown K, Dewey K, Allen L. *Complementary Feeding of Young Children in Developing Countries: A Review of Current Scientific Knowledge.* Geneva: WHO, 1998, pp. 30–32.[7]

Brown 1991

a. Brown KH. The relationship between diarrhoeal prevalence and growth of poor infants varies with their age and usual energy intake (abstract). *FASEB J* 1991;5:A1079.[86]

b. Brown K, Dewey K, Allen L. *Complementary Feeding of Young Children in Developing Countries: A Review of Current Scientific Knowledge.* Geneva: WHO, 1998, pp. 30–32.[7]

Castillo 1996

Castillo C, Atalah E, Riumallo J, Castro R. Breast-feeding and the nutritional status of nursing children in Chile. *Bull PAHO* 1996;30:125–133.[68]

Cohen 1994 (first Honduras trial)

a. Cohen RJ, Brown KH, Canahuati J, Rivera LL, Dewey KG. Effects of age of introduction of complementary foods on infant breast milk intake, total energy intake, and growth: a randomised intervention study in Honduras. *Lancet* 1994; 344:288–293.[63]

b. Cohen RJ, Brown KH, Canahuati J, Rivera LL, Dewey KG. Determinants of growth from birth to 12 months among breast-fed Honduran infants in relation to age of introduction of complementary foods. *Pediatrics* 1995;96:504–510.[69]

c. Dewey KG, Cohen RJ, Rivera LL, Canahuati J, Brown KH. Do exclusively breast-fed infants require extra protein? *Pediatr Res* 1996;39:303–307.[72]

d. Dewey KG, Cohen RJ, Rivera LL, Canahuati J, Brown KH. Effects of age at introduction of complementary foods to breast-fed infants on duration of lactational amenorrhea in Honduran women. *Am J Clin Nutr* 1997;65:1403–1409.[71]

e. Dewey KG, Cohen RJ, Rivera LL, Brown KH. Effects of age of introduction of complementary foods on iron status of breast-fed infants in Honduras. *Am J Clin Nutr* 1998;67:878–884.[71]

f. Dewey KG, Cohen RJ, Brown KH, Rivera LL. Effects of exclusive breastfeeding for four versus six months on maternal nutritional status and infant motor development: results of two randomized trials in Honduras. *J Nutr* 2001;131:262–267.[85]

Dewey 1999 (second Honduras trial)

a. Dewey KG, Cohen RJ, Rivera LL, Brown KH. Effects of age of introduction of complementary foods on micronutrient status of term, low-birthweight, breastfed infants in Honduras. *FASEB J* 1998; 12:A648.[70]

b. Dewey KG, Cohen J, Brown KH, Rivera LL. Age of introduction of complementary foods and growth of term, low-birth-weight, breast-fed infants: a randomized intervention study in Honduras. *Am J Clin Nutr* 1999;69:679–686.[64]

c. Dewey KG, Cohen RJ, Brown KH, Rivera LL. Effects of exclusive breastfeeding for four versus six months on maternal nutritional status and infant motor development: results of two randomized trials in Honduras. *J Nutr* 2001;131:262–267.[85]

Huffman 1987

Huffman SL, Ford K, Allen HA, Streble P. Nutrition and fertility in Bangladesh: breastfeeding and post partum amenorrhoea. *Population Studies* 1987; 41:447–462.[84]

Simondon 1997

Simondon KB, Simondon F. Age at introduction of complementary food and physical growth from 2 to 9 months in rural Senegal. *Eur J Clin Nutr* 1997; 51:703–707.[80]

Developed countries

Åkeson 1996

a. Åkeson PMK, Axelsson IE, Raiha NCR. Human milk and standard infant formula together with high quality supplementary foods is sufficient for normal growth during infancy. *Pediatr Res* 1996;39(Suppl): 313A.[81]

b. Åkeson PMK, Axelsson IE, Raiha NCR. Growth and nutrient intake in three- to twelve-month-old infants fed human milk or formulas with varying protein concentrations. *J Pediatr Gastroenterol Nutr* 1998; 26:1–8.[67]

c. Åkeson PMK, Axelsson IE, Raiha NCR. Protein and amino acid metabolism in three-to twelve-month-old infants fed human milk or formulas with varying protein concentrations. *J Pediatr Gastroenterol Nutr* 1998;26:297–304.[73]

Duncan 1993

Duncan B, Ey J, Holberg CJ, Wright AL, Martinez FD, Taussig LM. Exclusive breast-feeding for at least 4 months protects against otitis media. *Pediatrics* 1993; 91:867–872.[74]

Heinig 1993

Heinig MJ, Nommsen LA, Peerson JM, Lonnerdal B, Dewey KG. Intake and growth of breast-fed and formula-fed infants in relation to the timing of introduction of complementary foods: the DARLING study. *Acta Paediatr Scand* 1993;82:999–1006.[62]

Kajosaari 1983

a. Kajosaari M, Saarinen UM. Prophylaxis of atopic disease by six months' total solid food elimination. Evaluation of 135 exclusively breast-fed infants of atopic families. *Acta Paediatr Scand* 1983;72:411–414.[75]

b. Kajosaari M. Atopy prophylaxis in high-risk infants. Prospective 5-year follow-up study of children with six months exclusive breastfeeding and solid food elimination. *Adv Exp Med Biol* 1991;453–458.[77]

c. Kajosaari M. Atopy prevention in childhood: the role of diet: prospective 5-year follow-up of high-risk infants with six months exclusive breastfeeding and solid food elimination. *Pediatr Allerg Immunol* 1994;5:26–28.[76]

Kramer 2000

a. Kramer MS, Chalmers B, Hodnett ED, et al. Breastfeeding and infant growth: biology or bias *Pediatr Res* 2000;47:151A.[52]

b. Kramer MS, Chalmers B, Hodnett ED, et al. Promotion of Breastfeeding Intervention Trial (PROBIT): a cluster-randomized trial in the Republic of Belarus. In: Koletzko, Michaelsen KF, Hernell O, editors. *Short and Long Term Effects of Breast Feeding on Child Health.* New York: Kluwer Academic/Plenum Publishers, 2000, pp. 327–345.[53]

c. Kramer MS, Chalmers B, Hodnett ED, et al. Promotion of breastfeeding intervention trial (PROBIT): a randomized trial in the Republic of Belarus. *JAMA* 2001;285:413–420.[51]

Oddy 1999

Oddy W, Holt P, Sly P, Read A, Landau L, Stanley F, et al. Association between breast feeding and asthma in 6 year old children: findings of a prospective birth cohort study. *BMJ* 1999;319:815–819.[21]

Pisacane 1995

Pisacane A, de Vizla B, Valiante A, Vaccaro F, Russo M, Grillo G, et al. Iron status in breast-fed infants. *J Pediatr* 1995;127:429–431.[78]

WHO 1994

a. *WHO Working Group on Infant Growth. An evaluation of infant growth.* Doc WHO/NUT/94.8. Geneva: World Health Organization, 1994.[44]

b. Dewey KG, Peerson JM, Brown KH, Krebs NF, Michaaelsen KF, Persson LA, Salmenpera L, Whitehead RG, Yeung DL and the World Health Organization Working Group on Infant Growth. Growth of breast-fed infants deviates from current reference data: a pooled analysis of US, Canadian, and European data sets. *Pediatrics* 1995;96:495–503.[45]

c. WHO Working Group on Infant Growth. An evaluation of infant growth: the use and interpretation of anthropometry in infants. *Bull WHO* 1995;73:165–174.[88]

d. Brown K, Dewey K, Allen L. *Complementary feeding of young children in developing countries: a review of current scientific knowledge.* Geneva: WHO, 1998, pp. 28–29.[7]

WHO 1997

a. Frongillo EA Jr, de Onis M, Garza C, the World Health Organization Task Force on Methods for the Natural Regulation of Fertility. Effects of timing of complementary foods on postnatal growth. *FASEB J* 1997;11:A574.[82]

b. WHO Working Group on the Growth Reference Protocol and the WHO Task Force on Methods for the Natural Regulation of fertility. Growth of healthy infants and the timing, type and frequency of complementary foods. *Am J Clin Nutr* 2001. (In press).[83]

Review methods

Description of studies (see tables of included studies)

Methodologic quality of included studies (see tables of included studies)

Studies under consideration were evaluated for methodologic quality and appropriateness for inclusion without consideration of their results. The criteria for quality assessment were developed *a priori* and are presented below.

We used Cochrane criteria for assessing controlled clinical trials. As shown below, this method rates trials on three elements:

1. Adequacy of randomization and concealment:

    A. Randomized and concealed appropriately

    B. Randomized appropriately but concealment unclear from the description

    C. Not (or not reported as) randomized and/or inadequate concealment

2. Losses to follow-up and analysis:

    A. Used intention-to-treat (ITT) analysis, with losses to follow-up symmetrical and <15% in each group

    B. Symmetrical losses were ≥15%, but analysis was based on ITT

    C. Asymmetrical losses to follow-up despite use of ITT, or analysis not based on ITT

3. Measurement of outcome (outcome-specific):

    A. Blinding of observers or "objective" outcomes (e.g., measured weight)

    B. Nonblinding of observers for measurements that could be affected by bias (including length, head circumference, and self-reported outcomes)

The 5-point Jadad[89] scale was also used to examine the quality of randomized controlled trials. Details of the scale are as follows:

1. Was the study described as randomized (this includes the use of words such as randomly, random, and randomization)?

    a) not random or not mentioned (0)

    b) random, described, and inappropriate (0)

    c) random, not described (+1)

    d) random, described, and appropriate (+2)

2. Was the study described as double-blind?

    a) not double-blind (0)

    b) double-blind, described, and not appropriate (0)

    c) double-blind, not described (+1)

    d) double-blind, described, and appropriate (+2)

3. Was there a description of withdrawals and dropouts?

    Withdrawals (number and reasons) must be described by group to get 1 point

Observational (cohort, case-control, and cross-sectional studies) were assessed for control for confounding, losses to follow-up, and assessment of outcome as follows:

1. For growth and morbidity outcomes, control for confounding by socioeconomic status, water supply, sanitation facilities, parental height and weight, birth weight, and weight and length at 3 months (or age at which complementary feeding was introduced in the MBF group):

    A. Control for all (or almost all) pertinent confounders

    B. Partial control for some confounders

    C. No control for confounding

2. Losses to follow-up:

    A. Losses to follow-up were symmetrical and less than 15% in each group

    B. Losses were 15–25% and symmetrical

    C. Losses were >25%, asymmetrical, or not reported (and all cross-sectional studies)

3. Assessment of outcome (outcome-specific):

   A. Blinding of observers or "objective" outcomes (e.g., measured weight)

   B. Nonblinding of observers or measurements that could be affected by bias (including length, head circumference, and self-reported outcomes)

Quality assessments of all of the eligible studies were carried out independently by the two reviewers. Disagreements were resolved by consensus.

Data collection

Data were extracted independently by both reviewers, with disagreements resolved by consensus. Attempts were made to contact authors of all included studies to obtain additional data, resolve inconsistencies, and obtain additional methodologic details.

Data analysis

The studies were stratified according to study design (controlled trials vs observational studies), provenance (developing vs developed country), and timing of feeding comparison [(3–7 months vs "prolonged" (>6 months)]. One study,[82,83] based on a pooled analysis of 2 developed and 3 developing countries has been included with developed country studies because of the selection criteria (literate, educated, urban mothers) and the observed high infant growth rates. Analyses were carried out using the Review Manager 4.1 software for preparing Cochrane reviews. Effect measures are reported as the fixed-effect weighted mean difference (WMD) and its 95% confidence interval (CI) for continuous outcomes and the fixed-effect pooled relative risk (RR) and its 95% CI. For most continuous outcomes, a positive WMD denotes a higher (more favorable) value in the EBF group. All dichotomous outcomes are formulated as adverse; thus an RR <1 denotes that the EBF group had a lower risk of the outcome than the MBF group.

Table of included studies: Developing countries

Study	Methods	Participants	Interventions	Outcomes	Notes
Adair 1993 (P)	Design: prospective cohort Quality Assessment Control for confounding: A Follow-up: A Blinding: A for weight, B for length	1,204 Filipino infants	EBF = little or no nutritive foods or fluids other than BF for 6 months (n=370) MBF = BF with introduction of nutritive foods or liquids at 4 months (n=834)	Weight and length gain 4–6 months	Multivariate analysis did not affect outcome comparison, but data not presented.
Brown 1991 (P)	Design: prospective cohort Quality Assessment Control for confounding: B Follow-up: C Blinding: A for weight, B for length	36 poor, peri-urban Peruvian infants	EBF = little or no nutritive foods or fluids other than BF for 6 months (n=15) MBF = BF with introduction of nutritive foods and fluids at 4 months (n=21)	Weight and length gain 4–6 months	Multivariate analysis did not affect outcome comparison, but data not presented.
Castillo 1996 (P)	Design: cross-sectional Quality Assessment Control for confounding: C Follow-up: C Blinding: A for weight, B for length	1,122 Chilean children 3.0–5.9 months of age	EBF = BF only (unclear if water, juices, or other liquids permitted) (n=974) MBF = EBF for ≥2.9 months, then BF + solid food (n=148)	Low WAZ, LAZ; high WLZ	1. Cannot use data quantitatively, because prevalences, confidence intervals, and SEs not provided. 2. Low WAZ and LAZ defined as <-1, high WLZ as >+1.

Study	Methods	Participants	Interventions	Outcomes	Notes
Cohen 1994 (first Honduras trial) (P,U)	Design: controlled trial *Quality Assessment* Randomization: C Follow-up: C Blinding: A for weight and maternal postpartum weight loss; B for length, developmental milestones, and lactational amenorrhea *Jadad Scale* Randomization: 0/2 Double-blinding: 0/2 Withdrawals: 1/1 Total Jadad scale score: 1/5	141 Honduran infants of low-income families with poor sanitation	EBF = BF with no other liquids or solids until 6 months (n=50) MBF = introduction of complementary solid food at 4 months with either *ad libitum* nursing (SF) or maintenance of baseline nursing frequency (SF-M) (n=91)	Weight and length gain 4–6 and 6–12 months; WAZ, LAZ, and WLZ at 6 months; receipt of Fe supplements 6–9 months; hemoglobin and ferritin at 6 months; % of days with fever, cough, nasal congestion, nasal discharge, hoarseness, and diarrhea; age first crawled, age first sat from lying position, walking by 12 months; maternal postpartum weight loss 4–6 months; resumption of menses by 6 months	1. Nonrandom allocation. 2. Cluster allocation by week of birth, while analyses done at individual level. 3. Analysis not based on intention-to-treat. 4. SF-M and SF groups combined as MBF group.
Dewey 1999 (second Honduras trial) (P,U)	Design: controlled trial *Quality Assessment* Randomization: B Follow-up: C Blinding: A for weight, B for length *Jadad Scale* Randomization: 1/2 Double blinding: 0/2 Withdrawals: 1/1 Total Jadad scale score: 2/5	119 LBW Honduran term infants	EBF = BF with no other liquids or solids until 6 months (n=59) MBF = introduction of complementary solid food at 4 months with maintenance of baseline nursing frequency (n=60)	Weight and length gain 4–6 and 6–12 months; WAZ, LAZ, and WLZ at 6 months; plasma zinc concentration at 6 months; % of days with fever, cough, nasal congestion, nasal discharge, hoarseness, and diarrhea; age first crawled, age first sat from lying position, walking by 12 months; maternal postpartum weight loss 4–6 months; resumption of menses by 6 months	1. Cluster randomized by week of birth, while analyses done at individual level. 2. Analysis not based on intention-to-treat.
Huffman 1987 (P,U)	Design: prospective cohort *Quality Assessment* Control for confounding: C Follow-up: B Blinding: A	1,018 Bangladeshi women with live births	EBF = BF with no other liquids or solids for ≥7 months (n=647) MBF = EBF for 4 months with introduction of liquid or solid supplements before 7 months (n=371)	Duration of lactational amenorrhea	1. Over 95% of study women BF >16 months, so all MBF women assumed to continue BF ≥6 months. 2. Multivariate (Cox) regression controlled for maternal education, parity, religion, and weight, but reference group EBF <1 month.
Simondon 1997 (P,U)	Design: prospective cohort *Quality Assessment* Control for confounding: A for monthly weight and length gain 4–6 months; C for other outcomes Follow-up: B Blinding: A for weight and length	370 Senegalese infants recruited at 2–3 months	EBF = breast milk and water only until at least 6–7 months (n=154) MBF = breast milk, water, and introduction of complementary food between 4 and 7 months of age (n=216)	Monthly weight and length gain 4-6 and 6-9 months; WAZ, LAZ, and WLZ at 4–5, 6–7, and 9–10 months; mid-upper arm circumference at 4–5, 6–7, and 9–10 months	1. EBF = "very late" group, MBF = "early" and "late" groups combined. 2. Monthly weight and length gains 4–6 months based on multivariate control for maternal size and education and z-score at 2–3 months.

BF=breastfeeding, EBF=exclusive breastfeeding, MBF=mixed breastfeeding, P=published data; U=unpublished data

Table of included studies: Developed Countries

Study	Methods	Participants	Interventions	Outcomes	Notes
Åkeson 1996 (P)	Design: prospective cohort *Quality Assessment* Control for confounding: C Follow-up: C Blinding: A for weight and blood analyses, B for length	44 healthy Swedish infants EBF for the first 3 months	EBF = BF + <125 ml/day of formula for ≥6 months (n=26) MBF = EBF for ≥3 months, then BF ≥2 times/day + >125 ml/day of formula for ≥6 months (n=18)	Weight and length gain 4–8 months, 6–9, and 8–12 months; total and essential amino acid concentrations at 6 months	1. N's in tables not provided for weight and length. 2. Identical data for length gain for the two groups at 8–12 months: misprint?
Duncan 1993 (P,U)	Design: prospective cohort *Quality Assessment* Control for confounding: A Follow-up: B Blinding: B	279 healthy U.S. infants	EBF = EBF for ≥6 months (n=138) MBF = EBF for 4 months with introduction of formula or solid foods between 4 and 6 months (n=141)	Number of episodes of otitis media (OM), one or more episodes of OM, and frequent OM in first 12 months	
Heinig 1993 (P,U)	Design: prospective cohort *Quality Assessment* Control for confounding: C Follow-up: C Blinding: A for weight, B for length and sleeping time	60 healthy U.S. infants living in Davis, CA	EBF = BF ± ≤120 ml/day of other milk or formula for ≥12 months and no solids <6 months (n=19) MBF = BF ± ≤120 ml/day of other milk or formula for ≥12 months; solids introduced at 4–6 months (n=41)	Monthly weight and length gain at 6–9 and 9–12 months; total sleeping time at 9 months	1. Data on weight and length gain 4–6 months included in pooled analysis of WHO 1994. 2. No quantitative data presented on morbidity.
Kajosaari 1983 (P)	Design: prospective cohort *Quality Assessment* Control for confounding: B Follow-up: C Blinding: C	135 healthy Finnish infants of atopic parents	EBF = BF without cow milk-based formula; occasional water permitted; solids introduced at about 6 months (n=70) MBF = BF with introduction of solids at about 3 months (n=65)	Atopic eczema and food allergy at 1 year; any atopy, atopic eczema, pollen allergy, asthma, food allergy, and allergy to animal dander at 5 years	Discrepancy between 1- and 5-year follow-up reports regarding sample sizes per group (inverted from one report to the other).
Kramer 2000 (P,U)	Design: prospective cohort nested within randomized trial *Quality Assessment* Control for confounding: A Follow-up: A Blinding: A for weight, B for length and head circumference	3,483 healthy, term Belarussian infants	EBF = no liquids or solids other than breast milk for ≥6 months (n=621) MBF = EBF for 3 months with introduction of nonbreast milk liquids and/or solids by 6 months (n=2,862)	Monthly weight and length gain 3–6, 6–9, and 9–12 months; WAZ, LAZ, WLZ, and head circumference at 6, 9, and 12 months; death, occurrence of and hospitalization for gastrointestinal and respiratory infection, atopic eczema, and recurrent wheezing in first 12 months	Growth outcomes analyzed using multilevel regression controlling for geographic region, urban vs rural location, maternal education, and size or growth ≤3 months.
Oddy 1999 (P,U)	Design: prospective, cohort within randomized trial *Quality Assessment* Control for confounding: C Follow-up: A for 1-year outcomes, B for asthma at 6 years, C for skin prick tests at 6 years Blinding: B	510 Australian infants	EBF = no nonbreast milk or solids for ≥6 months (n=246) MBF = EBF for 4 months, with introduction of nonbreast milk and/or solids at 4–6 months (n=264)	Occurrence of and hospitalization for upper and lower respiratory tract infection and recurrent wheezing in first 12 months; asthma and positive skin-prick tests at 6 years	1. Published article includes multivariate control for confounders, but data included here are raw and unpublished. 2. Current asthma at 6 years defined as doctor-diagnosed + wheeze in previous year without a cold + receipt of asthma medication.

Study	Methods	Participants	Interventions	Outcomes	Notes
Pisacane 1995 (P)	Design: prospective cohort *Quality Assessment* Control for confounding: C Follow-up: C Blinding: A	30 term, appropriate-for-gestational-age Italian infants recruited at 6 months and BF for first year of life	EBF = BF only without any other fluids or solids for ≥7 months (n=9) MBF = EBF for 4-6 months with other foods introduced before 7 months (n=21)	Hemoglobin and serum ferritin concentrations at 12 months	
WHO 1994 (P,U)	Design: prospective cohort *Quality Assessment* Control for confounding: C Follow-up: C Blinding: A for weight, B for length	Pooled sample of healthy developed-country infants (n=358)	EBF = BF ± other liquids for ≥6 months (n=200) MBF = BF ± other liquids for ≥4 months with other milk ± solids introduced between 4 and 6 months (n=158)	Monthly weight and length gain 4–6 months	Multivariate control for initial weight and length, but data not presented.
WHO 1997 (P,U)	Design: prospective cohort *Quality Assessment* Control for confounding: A Follow-up: C Blinding: A for weight, B for length	Pooled sample of mid- to high-SES infants from 2 developed and 3 developing countries (n=556)	EBF = BF ± noncaloric liquids for ≥6 months (n=179) MBF = BF ± caloric liquids or solids introduced at 4–6 months (n=377)	Monthly weight and length gain 4–8 months	1. Multilevel regression used to control for maternal size and education and infant size and growth <4 months. 2. Large losses to follow-up; retained sample "similar" to full sample, but details not provided.

BF=breastfeeding, EBF=exclusive breastfeeding, MBF=mixed breastfeeding

Results

As discussed in the Review Methods, studies were stratified according to study design and provenance from developing vs developed countries. This resulted in three separate strata for considering the results of the studies located by the literature search: (1) controlled trials of exclusive vs mixed breastfeeding for 4–6 months from developing countries, (2) observational studies of exclusive vs mixed breastfeeding for 3–7 months from developing countries and (3) observational studies of exclusive vs mixed breastfeeding for 3–7 months from developed countries.

In accordance with conventional terminology used in Cochrane reviews, these strata are labeled below as "comparisons." Outcomes for each comparison are presented sequentially.

Comparison 1: Controlled trials of exclusive vs mixed breastfeeding for 4–6 months, developing countries

Two studies were found in this category, both from the same group of investigators and involving the same study setting (Honduras). The first of these studies, Cohen 1994, involved term infants unselected for birth weight but included 29 infants (19.9%) weighing <2500 g at birth. The second, Dewey 1999, was restricted to term infants weighing <2500 g at birth. The quality ratings of these two trials were not high for several reasons. First, in both trials, allocation was within clusters defined by weeks, rather than to individual women, yet the results were analyzed with individual women and infants as the units of analysis; any similarities in outcome within weeks (intracluster correlation) would tend to reduce the true effective sample size and thereby overestimate the precision (i.e., underestimate the variance) of the results. Second, the first trial allocated the weeks by alternation, rather than by strict randomization, thereby creating a potential for nonconcealment and uncontrolled confounding bias at enrollment (although there is no evidence that such bias actually occurred). Third, the published results were not based on analysis by intention-to-treat. Most of the subjects not analyzed in these two trials were truly lost to follow-up, however, rather than excluded for noncompliance; the latter were restricted to 4 subjects (3 in the exclusive breastfeeding group, 1 in the mixed breastfeeding group) in the first trial and 3 subjects (all 3 in the exclusive breastfeeding group) in the second trial. Moreover, the investigators have provided (unpublished) data on weight and length gain on 5 of the 9 dropouts in the second Honduran trial (3 of the 9 moved away before 6 months), thereby substantially reducing the potential for selection bias in the analysis of that trial.

Most importantly, despite the above-noted methodologic problems, these two trials are the only studies uncovered by our search that used an experimental design to specifically address the 4–6 months vs "about 6 months" controversy. Thus, at least with respect to bias due to known and unknown confounding variables, these trials are methodologically superior to any of the observational studies included in this review despite their methodologic imperfections. Furthermore, the investigators made a considerable effort to ensure compliance with the assigned allocation and to standardize the training of the observers who performed the anthropometric measurements, thereby reducing the random error (improving the precision) of these measurements. Finally, detailed comparisons between trial participants and eligible nonparticipants demonstrated no differences that would detract from the external validity (generalizability) of the trials' findings, at least for the specific type of setting where the study was conducted (an urban, low-income population in Honduras).

For all analyses, the two mixed breastfeeding groups (one of which was intended to maintain frequency of breastfeeding) in the first trial were combined for the purposes of this analysis. Monthly weight gain from 4 to 6 months was nonsignificantly slightly higher among infants whose mothers were assigned to continued exclusive breastfeeding [weighted mean difference (WMD) = +20.8 (95% CI -22.0 to +63.5) g/mo] (Outcome 1). Thus the 95% CI is statistically compatible with a weight gain only 22 g/mo lower in the EBF group, which represents approximately 5% of the mean and 15% of the SD for the monthly weight gain. Weight gain from 6 to 12 months (Outcome 2) was almost identical in the two groups [WMD = -2.6 (-25.9 to +20.6) g/mo].

For length gain from 4 to 6 months, the WMD was +1.0 mm/mo (-0.4 to +2.4 mm/mo); the lower confidence limit represents only 2% of the mean and 8% of the SD for monthly length gain (Outcome 3). As with weight gain, length gain from 6 to 12 months (Outcome 4) was nearly identical in the two groups [WMD = -0.4 (-1.0 to +0.2) mm/mo].

Weight-for-age, length-for-age, and weight-for-length z-scores at 6 months (Outcomes 5–7) were all nonsignificantly higher in the EBF group [WMD = +0.18 (-0.06 to +0.41), +0.11 (-0.11 to +0.33), and +0.09 (-0.13 to +0.31), respectively.

The impact of the small sample size of the two Honduran trials is evident when examining the risk of undernutrition, as represented by anthropometric z-scores <-2 at 6 months (Outcomes 8–10). For weight-for-age, the pooled relative risk (RR) was 2.14 (0.74–6.24), which is statistically compatible with a 6-fold increase in risk. The results were somewhat more reassuring for length-for-age [RR=1.18 (0.56–2.50)] but not for weight-for-length [RR = 1.38 (0.17–10.98)].

All hematologic results (Outcomes 11–19) are based on the first Honduras trial (Cohen 1994), since in the second trial (Dewey 1999, restricted to low birth weight infants), infants with low hemoglobin concentrations at 2 and 4 months were supplemented with iron. A nonsignificantly higher proportion of infants in the exclusively breastfed group received iron supplements from 6 to 9 months [RR = 1.20 (95% CI (0.91–1.58)] (Outcome 11). This is consistent with the significantly lower average hemoglobin concentration at 6 months in the exclusively breastfed group [difference = -5.0 (-8.5 to -1.5) g/L] (Outcome 12). A nonsignificantly higher proportion of exclusively breastfed infants had a hemoglobin concentration <110 g/L at 6 months [RR = 1.20 (0.91–1.58)] (Outcome 13). Similarly, mean plasma ferritin concentration was significantly lower at 6 months in the exclusively breastfed infants [difference = -18.9 (-37.3 to -0.5) mcg/L], with a RR for a low (<15 mcg/L) ferritin concentration of 2.93 (1.13–7.56) (Outcomes 17 and 19).

In the second trial, no significant effect was seen on the proportion of infants with a low zinc concentration (<70 mcg/dL) at 6 months [RR = 0.75 (0.43–1.33)] (Outcome 20).

In the pooled results from both Honduran trials, no significant difference was seen between the EBF and MBF groups for the percentage of days with fever, cough, or nasal congestion, nasal discharge, hoarseness, or diarrhea from 4 to 6 months (Outcomes 21–26), nor for fever, nasal congestion, or diarrhea from 6 to 12 months (Outcomes 27–29).

Again based on pooled results from both trials, mothers in the exclusively breastfed group reported that their infants crawled at an average of 0.8 (0.3 to 1.3) months sooner (Outcome 30). No difference was seen, however, in the mean age at which the infants were reported to have first sat from a lying position [WMD = -0.2 (-0.6 to +0.2) months] (Outcome 31). The results from the two Honduras trials differed with respect to maternal reports of walking by 12 months (Outcome 32), with a significantly lower proportion of exclusively breastfed infants reported as not having walked by 12 months in the first trial [RR = 0.66 (0.45–0.98)], but a nonsignificantly higher proportion not having done so in the second trial [RR = 1.12 (0.90–1.38)], with statistically significant ($P<.01$) heterogeneity between the two trials.

Mothers in the exclusively breastfed group (from the two trials combined) had a statistically significantly larger weight loss from 4 to 6 months [WMD = -0.42 (-0.82 to -0.02) kg] (Outcome 33). Women in the exclusively breastfed group were also nonsignificantly less likely to have resumed menses by 6 months postpartum [RR = 0.58 (0.33–1.03)]; the effect was statistically significant in the second Honduras trial when considered alone [RR = 0.35 (0.14–0.91)] (Outcome 34).

Comparison 2: Observational studies of exclusive vs mixed breastfeeding for 3–7 months, developing countries

The main concern in using an observational design to compare outcomes with EBF vs MBF is confounding due to differences in socioeconomic status, water and sanitation facilities, parental size (a proxy for genetic potential), and (perhaps most importantly) weight and length at the time complementary foods were first introduced in the mixed breastfeeding group. The latter source of confounding (i.e., by indication) will arise if poorly-growing infants are more likely to receive complementary foods.

Three cohort studies in this category from Peru (Brown 1991), the Philippines (Adair 1993), and Senegal (Simondon 1997) found no evidence of confounding by indication, Adair 1993 found no confounding by several other potential factors, and (in unpublished data provided by the authors) Simondon 1997 calculated adjusted means for weight and length gain from 4 to 6 months. Nonetheless, the inability of observational studies to control for subtle (and unknown) sources of confounding and selection bias suggests the need for cautious interpretation. All three studies reported on monthly weight gain from 4 to 6 months (Outcome 1). The WMD was -7.2 (-25.5 to +11.0) g/mo, a lower confidence limit compatible with a deficit of only 7% of the mean and <15% of the SD for monthly weight gain. The Simondon 1997 study also reported on monthly weight gain from 6 to 9 months [difference = -6.0 (-54.2 to +42.2) g/mo] (Outcome 2). All three studies reported on monthly length gain from 4–6 months (Outcome 3); the WMD was +0.4 (-0.3 to +1.2) mm/mo, a lower confidence limit statistically compatible with a reduced length gain in the EBF group of only 2% of the mean and 5% of the SD. The Simondon 1997 study also reported on monthly length gain from 6–9 months (Outcome 4), and again the results excluded all but a small reduction in the exclusively breastfed group [difference = +0.4 (-0.6 to +1.4) mm/mo].

The Simondon 1997 study also provided (unpublished) data on anthropometric z-scores and mid-upper arm circumference. EBF was associated with nonsignificantly higher WMD z-scores at 6–7 and 9–10 months: +0.13 (-0.09 to +0.35) and +0.09 (-0.15 to +0.33), respectively, for weight-for-age (Outcomes 5 and 6); +0.04 (-0.14 to +0.22) and +0.11 (-0.09 to +0.31), respectively, for length-for-age (outcomes 7 and 8); and +0.11 (-0.09 to +0.31) and +0.01 (-0.21 to +0.23), respectively, for weight-for-length (Outcomes 9 and 10). The relative risks for low (<-2) z-scores at 6–7 and 9–10 months were 0.92 (0.54–1.58) and 0.93 (0.64–1.36), respectively, for weight-for-age (Outcomes 11 and 12); 1.20 (0.57–2.53) and 1.21 (0.62–2.37), respectively, for length-for-age (Outcomes 13 and 14); and 0.42 (0.12–1.50) and 0.82 (0.39–1.72), respectively, for weight-for-length (Outcomes 15 and 16). Mid-upper arm circumference was nonsignificantly higher in the EBF group at both 6–7 and 9–10 months: WMD = +2.0 (-0.4 to +4.4) mm and +1.0 (-1.6 to +3.6) mm, respectively (Outcomes 17 and 18).

Huffman 1987 reported a longer median duration of lactational amenorrhea associated with EBF (for ≥7 months) vs MBF (16.1 vs 15.3 months, respectively), but means and SDs were not reported. In a multivariate (Cox) regression model adjusting for maternal education, parity, religion, and weight, EBF for ≥6 months was associated with a significantly longer time to resumption of menses vs EBF for <1 month, but no direct comparison was reported vs MBF.

Cross-sectional studies share all of the methodologic shortcomings of other observational designs (see above) plus one important additional one: selective loss to follow-up. In particular, children who die, are hospitalized, or are referred to a site other than the one under study may be more likely to experience morbidity or suboptimal growth. If such (unstudied) infants are more heavily represented in one of the feeding groups, the resulting comparison will be biased.

One large cross-sectional study from Chile (Castillo 1996) reported a similar risk of weight-for-age z-score <-1 and height-for-age z-score <-1 from 3–5 and 6–8 months in the two feeding groups, but the prevalences, confidence intervals, and standard errors for the reported prevalence ratios are not published, thus precluding any assessment of sampling variation.

Comparison 3: Observational studies of exclusive vs mixed breastfeeding for 3–7 months, developed countries

A pooled sample of breastfed infants from 7 studies in 6 developed countries (WHO 1994), a pooled analysis from 5 countries (2 developed, 3 developing, but in which study women were all literate and of middle to high socioeconomic status) (WHO 1997), a large cohort study nested within a randomized trial in Belarus (Kramer 2000), and a small study from Sweden (Åkeson 1996) reported on weight gain between 3 and 8 months. WHO 1997 and Kramer 2000 controlled for confounding by indication (size or growth in first 3–4 months) and other potential confounders using multilevel (mixed) regression analyses. Statistically significant (P=.02) heterogeneity was observed among the four studies, with considerably larger mean weight gains in both groups from Belarus and a slightly but significantly higher gain in the MBF group (Outcome 1). Because of this heterogeneity, the WMD of -12.5 (-23.5 to -1.4) g/mo should be interpreted with caution; even the lower 95% confidence limit of this estimate, however, is compatible with a lower weight gain in the EBF group of <4% of the mean and <15% of the SD for the Belarussian study. Moreover, given the large weight gains in both groups in the Belarussian study, the higher gain in the MBF group is not necessarily a beneficial outcome. Heinig 1993 and Kramer 2000 also reported on weight gain between 6 and 9 months (Outcome 2). Again, the results show significant heterogeneity (P=.04) but are dominated by the larger size of the Belarussian study. The pooled WMD was -2.3 (-16.9 to +12.4) g/mo. Åkeson 1996, Heinig 1993, and Kramer 2000 reported on weight gain from 8 to 12 months

(Outcome 3); the WMD was -1.8 (-16.7 to +13.1) g/mo, which excludes a reduced length gain in the EBF group of 5% of the mean and 10% of the SD for the Belarussian study.

For length gain at 3–8 months (Outcome 4), the studies again show significant (P<.01) heterogeneity. Kramer 2000 found a slightly but significantly lower length gain in the EBF group at 4–8 months [-1.1 (-1.7 to -0.5) mm/mo], whereas the pooled analysis yielded a WMD of -0.4 (-0.7 to 0.0) mm/mo; the lower confidence limit is statistically compatible with a reduced length gain of <4% of the mean and 10% of the SD for the Belarussian study. Heinig 1993 and Kramer 2000 also reported on length gain at 6–9 months [WMD = -0.4 (-1.0 to +0.1) mm/mo] (Outcome 5). For the 8–12 month period, the results show a slightly but significantly higher length gain in the EBF group [WMD = +0.9 (+0.3 to +1.4) mm/mo (Outcome 6).

Observational analyses from the Belarussian study (Kramer 2000) also include data on weight-for-age, length-for-age, and weight-for-length z-scores at 6, 9, and 12 months. Means in both the EBF and MBF groups were well above (+0.5 to +0.6) the reference values at all 3 ages. Nonetheless, the weight-for-age z-score was slightly but significantly lower in the EBF group at all 3 ages: WMD = -0.09 (-0.16 to -0.02) at 6 months, -0.10 (-0.18 to -0.02) at 9 months, and -0.09 (-0.17 to -0.01) at 12 months (Outcomes 7–9). Length-for-age z-scores were very close to the reference (0) at 6 and 9 months and slightly above the reference (0.15) at 12 months. Again, the EBF group had slightly but significantly (except at 12 months) lower values: WMD = -0.12 (-0.20 to -0.04) at 6 months, -0.14 (-0.22 to -0.06) at 9 months, and -0.02 (-0.10 to +0.06) at 12 months (Outcomes 10–12). Mean weight-for-length z-scores were high and rose (from about 0.65 to 0.80) from 6 to 12 months, with no significant differences between the EBF and MBF groups at any age: WMD = +0.02 (-0.07 to +0.11) at 6 months, +0.03 (-0.06 to +0.12) at 9 months, and -0.08 (-0.17 to +0.01) at 12 months (Outcomes 13–15).

The prevalence of low (<-2) z-scores did not differ significantly in the two Belarussian feeding groups for any of the three z-scores at any of the three ages, although the small number of infants with low z-scores provided low statistical power to detect such differences. RRs (and 95% CIs) for low weight-for-age were 0.92 (0.04–19.04) at 6 months, 1.52 (0.16–14.62) at 9 months and 1.15 (0.13–10.31) at 12 months (Outcomes 16–18). For length-for-age, the corresponding figures were 1.53 (0.84–2.78) at 6 months, 1.46 (0.80–2.64) at 9 months, and 0.66 (0.23–1.87) at 12 months (Outcomes 19–21). For weight-for-length, the figures were 0.31 (0.02–5.34) at 6 months, 1.14 (0.24–5.37) at 9 months, and 1.15 (0.13–10.31) at 12 months (Outcomes 22–24).

The Belarussian study also provided data on head circumference. No significant differences were observed at 6 months [WMD = -1.0 (-2.3 to +0.3) mm] (Outcome 25) or 9 months [+0.7 (-0.6 to +2.0) mm] (Outcome 26), but the EBF group had a slightly but significantly larger circumference at 12 months (Outcome 27): difference = +1.9 (+0.6 to +3.2) mm.

Heinig 1993 reported nearly identical sleeping time (729 vs 728 min/day) in the two groups (Outcome 28). Åkeson 1996 reported similar total amino acid and essential amino acid concentrations at 6 months of age in the two feeding groups (Outcomes 29 and 30). Both Kramer 2000 and a cohort study from Finland (Kajosaari 1983) reported an atopic eczema at one year (Outcome 31). The two studies showed statistically significant (P=.03) heterogeneity, with Kajosaari 1983 reporting a significantly reduced risk [RR = 0.40 (0.21–0.78)], but the larger Belarussian study finding a much lower absolute risk in both feeding groups and no risk reduction with EBF [RR = 1.00 (0.60–1.69)]. Although Kajosaari 1983 also reported a reduced risk of a history of food allergy (Outcome 32), double food challenges showed no significant risk reduction [RR = 0.77 (0.25–2.41)] (Outcome 33). Neither Oddy 1999 nor Kramer 2000 found a significant reduction in risk of recurrent (2 or more episodes) wheezing in the EBF group [pooled RR = 0.79 (0.49–1.28)] (Outcome 34). In the Kajosaari 1983 study, the reduction in risk of any atopy at 5 years (Outcome 35) in the EBF group was nonsignificant [RR = 0.68 (0.40–1.17)], and no reduction in risk was observed for atopic eczema [RR = 0.97 (0.50–1.89)] (Outcome 36). A reduction in risk of borderline significance was observed for pollen allergy at 5 years [RR = 0.53 (0.28–1.01)] (Outcome 37). Both Kajosaari 1983 and Oddy 1999 reported on risk of asthma at 5–6 years (Outcome 38); the pooled RR was 0.91 (0.61–1.36). Reduced risks of history of food allergy [RR = 0.61 (0.12–3.19)] (Outcome 39) and allergy to animal dander [RR = 0.81 (0.24–2.72)] at 5 years (Outcome 40) were far from achieving statistical significance. Oddy 1999 found no reduction in risk of a positive skin prick test at 6 years in the EBF group [RR = 0.99 (0.73–1.35)] (Outcome 41).

A small Italian study of hematologic outcomes at 12 months by Pisacane in 1995 reported a statistically significantly higher hemoglobin concentration [117 vs

109 g/L (95% CI for the difference = +4.0 to +12.0 g/L)] (Outcome 42), a nonsignificant reduction in anemia (hemoglobin <110 g/L) [RR = 0.12 (0.01–1.80)] (Outcome 43), a nonsignificantly higher ferritin concentration [WMD = +4.7 (-6.3 to +15.7 mcg/L)] (Outcome 44), and a nonsignificant reduction in the risk of low (<10 mcg/L) ferritin concentration [RR = 0.42 (0.12–1.54)] (Outcome 45) among infants in the exclusive breastfeeding group. Of note in this study is that the exclusive and mixed breastfeeding continued in both groups until at least 12 months (a criterion for selection into the Pisacane et al study[78]).

Kramer 2000 recorded only 1 and 2 deaths (Outcome 46) among the 621 and 2,862 Belarussian infants in the EBF and MBF groups, respectively [RR = 2.30 (0.21–25.37)]. The EBF had a significantly reduced risk of one or more episodes of gastrointestinal infection in the first 12 months of life [RR = 0.67 (0.46–0.97)] (Outcome 47), which was maintained in a multivariate mixed model controlling for geographic origin, urban vs rural location, maternal education, and number of siblings in the household [adjusted OR = 0.61 (0.41–0.93)]. No significant reduction in risk was observed for hospitalization for gastrointestinal infection, however [RR = 0.79 (0.42–1.49)] (Outcome 48). In the above-mentioned Australian cohort study, Oddy 1999 found no significant reduction of risk for one or more episodes of upper respiratory tract infection (Outcome 49) in the EBF group [RR = 1.07 (0.96–1.20)]. Neither Oddy 1999 nor Kramer 2000 found a significantly reduced risk of 2 or more such episodes [pooled RR = 0.91 (0.82–1.02)] (Outcome 50). Nor did Oddy 1999 find a significant reduction in risk of 4 or more episodes of upper respiratory infection [RR = 0.82 (0.52–1.29)] (Outcome 51) or of one or more episodes of lower respiratory tract infection [RR = 1.07 (0.86–1.33)] (Outcome 52). Kramer 2000 found a small and nonsignificant reduction in risk of 2 or more respiratory tract infections (upper and lower combined): RR = 0.90 (0.79–1.03) (Outcome 53). The combined crude results of Oddy 1999 and Kramer 2000 show a substantial and statistically significant reduction in risk for hospitalization for respiratory tract infection [pooled RR = 0.75 (0.60–0.94)], but the crude risk reduction in Kramer 2000 was nearly abolished and became statistically nonsignificant in a multivariate mixed model controlling for geographic region, urban vs rural location, maternal education and cigarette smoking, and number of siblings in the household [adjusted OR = 0.96 (0.71–1.30)] (Outcome 54).

In a study from Tucson, Arizona, Duncan et al (1993) reported no difference in the average number of episodes of acute otitis media in the first 12 months of life (Outcome 55) in the exclusive vs mixed breastfeeding groups (1.48 vs 1.52 episodes, respectively) (95% confidence interval for the difference = -0.49 to +0.41 episodes). Duncan 1993 and Kramer 2000 both found a slightly elevated risk for one or more episodes of otitis media [pooled RR = 1.28 (1.04–1.57)] (Outcome 56), but Duncan 1993 found a nonsignificant reduction in risk for frequent otitis media [RR = 0.81 (0.43–1.52)] (Outcome 57).

Discussion

Summary of findings

Neither the controlled clinical trials nor the observational studies (predominantly cohort studies) from either developing or developed countries suggest that infants who continue to be exclusively breastfed for 6 months show deficits in weight or length gain from 3 to 7 months or thereafter. Owing to the large sample sizes required to detect small effects on the incidence of low (<-2) anthropometric z-scores, however, the data are insufficient to rule out a small increase in risk of undernutrition with exclusive breastfeeding for 6 months.

The large Belarussian study (Kramer 2000) found a significant reduction in risk of one or more episodes of gastrointestinal infection. No other significant reduction in infectious morbidity has been demonstrated, and the combined data from Finland, Australia, and Belarus do not suggest a protective effect against short- or long-term atopic outcomes.

The data are limited with respect to iron status, but the controlled trials from Honduras suggest that, at least in developing country settings where maternal iron status (and thus newborn iron stores) may be suboptimal, exclusive breastfeeding without iron supplementation may compromise hematologic status by 6 months of age. The reasons for the superior hematologic status reported in Italian infants exclusively breastfed for ≥7 months are unclear.

Data from the two Honduran trials and the Bangladeshi cohort study suggest that exclusive breastfeeding through 6 months is associated with delayed resumption of menses, at least in settings with high breastfeeding frequency. The more prolonged lactational amenorrhea represents an additional advantage of continued exclusive breastfeeding in developing country settings.

The two Honduran trials also found prolonged exclusive breastfeeding to be associated with more rapid maternal postpartum weight loss. Such an effect would be an additional benefit if it were generalizable to developed country settings where gestational weight gains and postpartum weight retention are high, but would be a disadvantage if it applied to undernourished women in developing countries.

In the two Honduran trials, mothers allocated to the prolonged exclusive breastfeeding group reported that their infants crawled at a significantly younger age. No such difference was seen, however, in the age at which the infants first sat from lying position, and the results for walking by 12 months differed in the two trials. The inconsistency of these results, coupled with the potential for biased maternal reporting due to nonblinding, suggest the need for cautious interpretation and further study.

Implications for future research

The investigators involved in the two Honduran trials took a step in the right direction when they opted for an experimental design to overcome problems with confounding (particularly confounding by indication) and selection bias inherent in observational designs. The results of observational studies from developing countries are consistent with the results of the two Honduran trials, especially with respect to growth. Nonetheless, the small number of studies and of infants studied, as well as uncertainty about the net direction and magnitude of potential biases, underscore the need for further research, particularly to rule out a small increase in risk of undernutrition.

It would seem prudent, therefore, to undertake larger, truly randomized trials of exclusive breastfeeding for 6 months to exclude increased risks of malnutrition (in developing countries), and to confirm or undermine the findings on infectious morbidity and neuromotor development. Because of the strong potential for contamination (similar practices among women who interact with one another), cluster randomization by clinic or even community may well be the preferred research design strategy. Longer-term impacts on intelligence, behavior, blood pressure, growth, and atopic disease are also worth pursuing.

Conclusion

We found no objective evidence of a "weanling's dilemma." Besides their reduced morbidity due to gastrointestinal infection, infants breastfed exclusively for 6 or more months had no observable deficits in growth, and their mothers were more likely to remain amenorrheic for 6 months postpartum. No benefits of introducing complementary foods between 4 and 6 months have been demonstrated, with the exception of improved iron status in one developing country setting (Honduras). Since the latter benefit can be achieved more effectively by medicinal iron supplementation (e.g., vitamin drops), it does not appear to justify incurring the adverse effects of liquid or solid food supplementation on infectious morbidity, and lactational amenorrhea.

Thus, with the caveat that individual infants must still be managed individually, so that insufficient growth or other adverse outcomes are not ignored and appropriate interventions are provided, the available evidence demonstrated no apparent risks in recommending, as a general policy, exclusive breastfeeding for the first 6 months of life in both developing and developed country settings. Large, rigorous cluster-randomized trials should help resolve residual uncertainties about the possible advantages and disadvantages of such a policy.

References

1. Waterlow J, Thomson A. Observations on the adequacy of breast-feeding. *Lancet* 1979; ii:238–241.

2. Whitehead R, Paul A. Growth charts and the assessment of infant feeding practices in the western world and in developing countries. *Early Hum Dev* 1984; 9:187–207.

3. FAO/WHO. Energy and protein requirements. 1973; Rome: FAO. 52: FAO Nutrition meetings.

4. Whitehead R, Paul A. Infant growth and human milk requirements. *Lancet* 1981; 161–163.

5. Garza C, Butte N. Energy intakes of human milk-fed infants during the first year. *J Pediatr* 1990; 117:S124–S131.

6. Butte N. Energy requirements of infants. *Eur J Clin Nutr* 1996; (suppl) 50:24–36.

7. Brown K, Dewey K, Allen L. *Complementary Feeding of Young Children in Developing Countries: A Review of Current Scientific Knowledge*. Geneva: WHO, 1998.

8. World Health Organization. Energy and protein requirements. 1985; Report of a Joint FAO/WHO/UNU Expert Consultation ed., Geneva: *Technical Report Series*, 724.

9. Rowland M, Barrell R, Whitehead R. Bacterial contamination in traditional Gambian weaning foods. *Lancet* 1978; i:136–138.

10. Rowland M. The weanling's dilemma: Are we making progress? *Acta Paediatr Scand* 1986; (suppl) 323:33-42.

11. WHO Collaborative Study Team on the Role of Breastfeeding on the Prevention of Infant Mortality. Effect of breastfeeding on infant and child mortality due to infectious diseases in less developed countries: a pooled analysis. *Lancet* 2001; 355:451–455.

12. Anandaiah R, Choe M. *Are the WHO guidelines on breastfeeding appropriate for India?* National Family Health Survey Subject Reports, Number 16 2000.

13. Howie P, Forsyth J, Ogston S, Clark A, du V Florey C. Protective effect of breast feeding against infection. *Br Med J* 1990; 300:11–16.

14. Cunningham A, Jelliffe D, Jelliffe E. Breast-feeding and health in the 1980's: a global epidemiologic review. *J Pediatr* 1991; 118:659–666.

15. Beaudry M, Dufour R, Marcoux S. Relation between infant feeding and infections during the first six months of life. *J Pediatr* 1995; 126:191–197.

16. Dewey K, Heinig M, Nommsen-Rivers L. Differences in morbidity between breast-fed and formula fed infants. *J Pediatr* 1995; 126:696–702.

17. Raisler J, Alexander C, O'Campo P. Breast-feeding and infant illness: a dose-response relationship? *Am J Public Health* 1999; 89:25–30.

18. Ford R, Taylor B, Mitchell E, Enright S, Stewart A, Becroft D, et al. Breastfeeding and the risk of sudden infant death syndrome. *Int J Epidemiol* 1993; 22:885–890.

19. Saarinen U, Backman A, Kajosaari M, Simes M. Prolonged breast-feeding as prophylaxis for atopic disease. *Lancet* 1979; ii:163–166.

20. Hide D, Guyer B. Clinical manifestations of allergy related to breast and cow's milk feeding. *Arch Dis Child* 1981; 56:172–175.

21. Oddy W, Holt P, Sly P, Read A, Landau L, Stanley F, et al. Association between breast feeding and asthma in 6 year old children: findings of a prospective birth cohort study. *BMJ* 1999; 319:815–819.

22. Lucas A, Morley R, Cole T, et al. Breast milk and subsequent intelligence quotient in children born preterm. *Lancet* 1992; 339:261–264.

23. Lanting C, Fidler V, Huisman M, et al. Neurological differences between 9-year old children fed breast-milk or formula-milk as babies. *Lancet* 1994; 344:1319–1322.

24. Horwood L, Fergusson D. Breastfeeding and later cognitive and academic outcomes. *Pediatrics* 1998; 101:e9.

25. Anderson J, Johnstone B, Remley D. Breast-feeding and cognitive development: a meta-analysis. *Am J Clin Nutr* 1999; 70:525–535.

26. Vestergaard M, Obel C, Henriksen T, Sørensen H, Skajaa E, Østergaard J. Duration of breastfeeding and developmental milestones during the latter half of infancy. *Acta Paediatr* 1999; 88:1327–1332.

27. San Giovanni J, Berkey C, Dwyer J, Colditz G. Dietary essential fatty acids, long chain polyunsaturated fatty acids, and visual resolution acuity in healthy fullterm infants: a systematic review. *Early Hum Dev* 2000; 57:165–188.

28. San Giovanni J, Parra-Cabrera S, Colditz G, Berkey C, Dwyer J. Meta-analysis of dietary essential fatty acids and long chain polyunsaturated fatty acids as they relate to visual resolution acuity in healthy preterm infants. *Pediatrics* 2000; 105:1292–1298.

29. Kramer M. Do breast-feeding and delayed introduction of solid foods protect against subsequent obesity? *J Pediatr* 1981; 98:883–887.

30. von Kries R, Koletzko B, Sauerwald T, von Mutius E, Barnert D, Grunert V, et al. Breast feeding and obesity: cross sectional study. *BMJ* 1999; 319:147–150.

31. Gillman M, Rifas-Shiman S, Camargo C, Berkey C, Frazier A, Rockett H, et al. Risk of overweight among adolescents who were breastfed as infants. *JAMA* 2001; 285:2461–2467.

32. Mayer E, Hamman R, Gay E, et al. Reduced risk of IDDM among breastfed children. *Diabetes* 1988; 37:1625–1632.

33. Gerstein H. Cow's-milk exposure and type-I diabetes mellitus: a critical review of the clinical literature. *Diabetes Care* 1994; 17:13–19.

34. Koletzko S, Sherman P, Corey M, et al. Role of infant feeding practices in development of Crohn's disease in childhood. *Br Med J* 1989; 298:1617–1618.

35. Davis M, Savitz D, Graubard B. Infant feeding and childhood cancer. *Lancet* 1988; 2:365–368.

36. Davis M. Review of the evidence for an association between infant feeding and childhood cancer. *Int J Cancer* 1998; (suppl) 11:29–33.

37. Chilvers C. Breastfeeding and risk of breast cancer in young women. *Br Med J* 1993; 307:17–20.

38. Brinton L, Potischman N, Swanson C, et al. Breastfeeding and breast cancer risk. *Cancer Causes and Control* 1995; 6:199–208.

39. Enger S, Ross R, Henderson B, Bernstein L. Breastfeeding history pregnancy experience and risk of breast cancer. *Br J Cancer* 1997; 76:118–123.

40. Rosenblatt K, Thomas D. Lactation and the risk of epithelial ovarian cancer. *Int J Epidemiol* 1993; 22:192–197.

41. Alderman B, Weiss N, Daling J, et al. Reproductive history and postmenopausal risk of hip and forearm fracture. *Am J Epidemiol* 1986; 124:262–267.

42. Melton L, Bryant S, Wahner H. Influence of breastfeeding and other reproductive factors in bone mass later in life. *Osteoporosis Int* 1993; 3:76–83.

43. Cummings R, Klineberg R. Breastfeeding and other reproductive factors and the risk of hip fractures in elderly women. *Int J Epidemiol* 1993; 22:684–691.

44. WHO Working Group on Infant Growth. *An evaluation of infant growth*. Geneva: World Health Organization, 1994.

45. Dewey K, Peerson J, Brown K, Krebs N, Michaelsen K, Persson L, et al. Growth of breast-fed infants deviates from current reference data: a pooled analysis of US, Canadian, and European data sets. *Pediatrics* 1995; 96:495–503.

46. Nielsen G, Thomsen B, Michaelsen K. Influence of breastfeeding and complementary food on growth between 5 and 10 months. *Acta Paediatr* 1998; 87:911–917.

47. Hediger M, Overpeck M, Ruan W, Troendle J. Early infant feeding and growth status of US-born infants and children aged 4–71 mo: analyses from the third National Health and Nutrition Examination Survey, 1988–1994. *Am J Clin Nutr* 2000; 72:159–167.

48. Haschke F, van't Hof M, Euro-growth study groups. Euro-Growth references for breast-fed boys and girls: influence of breast-feeding and solids on growth until 36 months of age. *J Pediatr Gastroenterol Nutr* 2000; 31:S60–S71.

49. de Onis M, Garza C, Habicht J. Time for a new growth reference. *Pediatrics* 1997; 100:E8.

50. WHO Working Group on the Growth Reference Protocol and WHO Task Force on Methods for the Natural Regulation of Fertility. Growth patterns of breastfed infants in seven countries. *Acta Paediatr* 2000; 89:215–222.

51. Kramer M, Chalmers B, Hodnett E, Sevkovskaya Z, Dzikovich I, Shapiro S, et al. Promotion of

breastfeeding intervention trial (PROBIT): A randomized trial in the Republic of Belarus. *JAMA* 2001; 285:413–420.

52. Kramer M, Chalmers B, Hodnett E. Breastfeeding and infant growth: biology or bias? *Pediatr Res* 2000; 47:151A.

53. Kramer MS, Chalmers B, Hodnett ED, et al. Promotion of Breastfeeding Intervention Trial (PROBIT): a cluster-randomized trial in the Republic of Belarus. In: Koletzko, Michaelsen KF, Hernell O, editors. *Short and Long Term Effects of Breast Feeding on Child Health*. New York: Kluwer Academic/Plenum Publishers, 2000, pp. 327–345.

54. World Health Organization. Nutrition: Information and attitudes among health personnel about early infant-feeding practices. WHO *Wkly Epidem* 1995; 70:117–120.

55. United Nations Children's Fund. *Facts for Life*. Wallingford: P&LA, 1993.

56. Lutter C. Length of exclusive breastfeeding: linking biology and scientific evidence to a public health recommendation. *J Nutr* 2000; 130:1335–1338.

57. Committee on Nutrition, American Academy of Pediatrics. *Pediatric Nutrition Handbook*. 4th ed. Elk Grove Village, Illinois: American Academy of Pediatrics, 1998.

58. Hill A. *A Short Textbook of Medical Statistics*. London: Hodder & Stoughton, 1977, p.27.

59. Sauls H. Potential effect of demographic and other variables in studies comparing morbidity of breast-fed and bottle-fed infants. *Pediatrics* 1979; 64:523–527.

60. Miettinen O. The need for randomization in the study of intended effects. *Stat Med* 1983; 2:267–271.

61. Bauchner H, Leventhal J, Shapiro E. Studies of breast-feeding and infections: How good is the evidence? *JAMA* 1986; 256:887–892.

62. Heinig M, Nommsen L, Peerson J, Lonnerdal B, Dewey K. Intake and growth of breast-fed and formula-fed infants in relation to the timing of introduction of complementary foods: the DARLING study. *Acta Paediatr Scand* 1993; 82:999–1006.

63. Cohen R, Brown K, Canahuati J, Rivera L, Dewey K. Effects of age of introduction of complementary foods on infant breast milk intake, total energy intake, and growth: a randomized intervention study in Honduras. *Lancet* 1994; 344:288–293.

64. Dewey K, Cohen R, Brown K, Rivera L. Age of introduction of complementary foods and growth of term, low-birthweight, breast-fed infants: a randomized intervention study in Honduras. *Am J Clin Nutr* 1999; 69:679–686.

65. Frongillo EJr, Habicht J-P. Investigating the weanling's dilemma: lessons from Honduras. *Nutrition Reviews* 1997; 55:390–395.

66. *Indicators for Assessing Breast-Feeding Practices*. Geneva, Switzerland: World Health Organization. WHO Document WHO/CDD/SER 1991; 91:14.

67. Åkeson P, Axelsson I, Raiha N. Growth and nutrient intake in three-to-twelve-month-old infants fed human milk or formulas with varying protein concentrations. *J Pediatr Gastroenterol Nutr* 1998; 26:1–8.

68. Castillo C, Atalah E, Riumallo J, Castro R. Breastfeeding and the nutritional status of nursing children in Chile. *Bull PAHO* 1996; 30:125–133.

69. Cohen R, Brown K, Canahuati J, Rivera L, Dewey K. Determinants of growth from birth to 12 months among breast-fed Honduran infants in relation to age of introduction of complementary foods. *Pediatrics* 1995; 96:504–510.

70. Dewey K, Cohen R, Rivera L, Brown K. Effects of age of introduction of complementary foods on micronutrient status of term, low-birthweight, breastfed infants in Honduras. *FASEB J* 1998; 12:A648.

71. Dewey K, Cohen R, Rivera L, Brown K. Effects of age introduction of complementary foods on iron status of breast-fed infants in Honduras. *Am J Clin Nutr* 1998; 67:878–884.

72. Dewey K, Cohen R, Rivera L, Canahuati J, Brown K. Do exclusively breast-fed infants require extra protein? *Pediatr Res* 1996; 39:303–307.

73. Åkeson P, Axelsson I, Raiha N. Protein and amino acid metabolism in three-to-twelve-month-old infants fed human milk or formulas with varying protein concentrations. *J Pediatr Gastroenterol Nutr* 1998; 26:297–304.

74. Duncan B, Ey J, Holberg C, Wright A, Martinez F, Taussig L. Exclusive breast-feeding for at least 4 months protects against otitis media. *Pediatrics* 1993; 91:867–872.

75. Kajosaari M, Saarinen U. Prophylaxis of atopic disease by six months' total solid food elimination. Evaluation of 135 exclusively breast-fed infants of

atopic families. *Acta Paediatr Scand* 1983; 72:411–414.

76. Kajosaari M. Atopy prevention in childhood: the role of diet: a prospective 5-year follow-up of high-risk infants with six months exclusive breastfeeding and solid food elimination. *Pediatr Allerg Immunol* 1994; 5:26–28.

77. Kajosaari M. Atopy prophylaxis in high-risk infants. Prospective 5-year follow-up study of children with six months exclusive breastfeeding and solid food elimination. *Adv Exp Med Biol* 1991; 310:453–458.

78. Pisacane A, de Vizia B, Valiante A, Vaccaro F, Russo M, Grillo G, et al. Iron status in breast-fed infants. *J Pediatr* 1995; 127:429–431.

79. Adair L, Popkin B, Vanderslice J, Akin J, Guilkey D, Black R, et al. Growth dynamics during the first two years of life: a prospective study in teh Phillipines. *Eur J Clin Nutr* 1993; 47:42–51.

80. Simondon K, Simondon F. Age at introduction of complementary food and physical growth from 2 to 9 months in rural Senegal. *Eur J Clin Nutr* 1997; 51:703–707.

81. Åkeson P, Axelsson I, Raiha N. Human milk and standard infant formula together with high quality supplementary foods is sufficient for normal growth during infancy. *Pediatr Res* 1996; 39 (Suppl):313A.

82. Frongillo EJ, de Onis M, Garza C. The World Health Organization Task Force on Methods for the Natural Regulation of Fertility. Effects of timing of complementary foods on post-natal growth. *FASEB Journal* 1997; 11:A574.

83. WHO Working Group on the Growth Reference Protocol and the WHO Task Force on Methods for the Natural Regulation of fertility. Growth of healthy infants and the timing, type and frequency of complementary foods. *Am J Clin Nutr* 2001. (In press).

84. Huffman S, Ford K, Allen H, Streble P. Nutrition and fertility in Bangladesh: breastfeeding and post partum amenorrhoea. *Population Studies* 1987; 41:447–462.

85. Dewey K, Cohen R, Brown K, Rivera L. Effects of exclusive breastfeeding for four versus six months on maternal nutritional status and infant motor development: results of two randomized trials in Honduras. *J Nutr* 2001; 131:262–267.

86. Brown K. The relationship between diarrhoeal prevalence and growth of poor infants varies with their age and usual energy intake (abstract). *FASEB J* 1991; 5:A1079.

87. Dewey K, Cohen R, Rivera L, Canahuati J, Brown K. Effects of age at introduction of complementary foods to breast-fed infants on duration of lactational amenorrhea in Honduran women. *Am J Clin Nutr* 1997; 65:1403–1409.

88. WHO Working Group on Infant Growth. An evaluation of infant growth: the use and interpretation of anthropometry in infants. *Bull WHO* 1995; 73:165–174.

89. Jadad A, Moore R, Carroll D, Jenkinson C, Reynolds J, Gavaghan D, et al. Assessing the quality of reports of randomized clinical trials: is blinding necessary? *Controlled Clinical Trials* 1996; 17:1–12.

ANNEX 1

Comparison 01: Exclusive vs mixed breastfeeding 4–6 months, developing countries, controlled trials

Comparison: 01 Exclusive vs mixed breastfeeding 4-6 months, developing countries, controlled trials
Outcome: 01 Monthly weight gain from 4-6 months (g/mo)

Study	EBF n	mean(sd)	MBF n	mean(sd)	WMD (95%CI Fixed)	Weight %	WMD (95%CI Fixed)
Cohen 1994	50	546.00(178.00)	91	514.00(154.00)		53.2	32.00[-26.61,90.61]
Dewey 1999	63	511.50(173.00)	61	503.50(182.00)		46.8	8.00[-54.54,70.54]
Total(95%CI)	113		152			100.0	20.78[-21.99,63.54]

Test for heterogeneity chi-square=0.30 df=1 p=0.58
Test for overall effect z=0.95 p=0.3

-100 -50 0 50 100
Favours MBF   Favours EBF

Comparison: 01 Exclusive vs mixed breastfeeding 4-6 months, developing countries, controlled trials
Outcome: 02 Monthly weight gain from 6-12 months (g/mo)

Study	EBF n	mean(sd)	MBF n	mean(sd)	WMD (95%CI Fixed)	Weight %	WMD (95%CI Fixed)
Cohen 1994	47	212.81(91.85)	87	216.55(84.54)		53.7	-3.74[-35.44,27.96]
Dewey 1999	51	221.49(87.20)	48	222.80(86.18)		46.3	-1.31[-35.47,32.85]
Total(95%CI)	98		135			100.0	-2.62[-25.85,20.62]

Test for heterogeneity chi-square=0.01 df=1 p=0.92
Test for overall effect z=0.22 p=0.8

-100 -50 0 50 100
Favours MBF   Favours EBF

Comparison: 01 Exclusive vs mixed breastfeeding 4-6 months, developing countries, controlled trials
Outcome: 03 Monthly length gain 4-6 months (cm/mo)

Study	EBF n	mean(sd)	MBF n	mean(sd)	WMD (95%CI Fixed)	Weight %	WMD (95%CI Fixed)
Cohen 1994	50	1.95(0.60)	91	1.90(0.55)		48.8	0.05[-0.15,0.25]
Dewey 1999	63	2.30(0.65)	61	2.15(0.45)		51.2	0.15[-0.05,0.35]
Total(95%CI)	113		152			100.0	0.10[-0.04,0.24]

Test for heterogeneity chi-square=0.49 df=1 p=0.49
Test for overall effect z=1.41 p=0.16

-.5 -.25 0 .25 .5
Favours MBF   Favours EBF

Comparison: 01 Exclusive vs mixed breastfeeding 4-6 months, developing countries, controlled trials
Outcome: 04 Monthly length gain 6-12 months (cm/mo)

Study	EBF n	mean(sd)	MBF n	mean(sd)	WMD (95%CI Fixed)	Weight %	WMD (95%CI Fixed)
Cohen 1994	47	1.19(0.18)	87	1.20(0.24)		64.3	-0.01[-0.08,0.06]
Dewey 1999	51	1.14(0.24)	48	1.23(0.25)		35.7	-0.09[-0.19,0.01]
Total(95%CI)	98		135			100.0	-0.04[-0.10,0.02]

Test for heterogeneity chi-square=1.69 df=1 p=0.19
Test for overall effect z=1.31 p=0.19

-.5 -.25 0 .25 .5
Favours MBF   Favours EBF

Comparison: 01 Exclusive vs mixed breastfeeding 4-6 months, developing countries, controlled trials
Outcome: 05 Weight-for-age z-score at 6 months

Study	EBF n	mean(sd)	MBF n	mean(sd)	WMD (95%CI Fixed)	Weight %	WMD (95%CI Fixed)
Cohen 1994	50	0.15(1.03)	91	-0.09(0.92)		46.9	0.24[-0.10,0.58]
Dewey 1999	59	-0.75(1.02)	60	-0.87(0.75)		53.1	0.12[-0.20,0.44]
Total(95%CI)	109		151			100.0	0.18[-0.06,0.41]
Test for heterogeneity chi-square=0.25 df=1 p=0.62							
Test for overall effect z=1.47 p=0.14							

-1 -.5 0 .5 1
Favours MBF   Favours EBF

Comparison: 01 Exclusive vs mixed breastfeeding 4-6 months, developing countries, controlled trials
Outcome: 06 Length-for-age z-score at 6 months

Study	EBF n	mean(sd)	MBF n	mean(sd)	WMD (95%CI Fixed)	Weight %	WMD (95%CI Fixed)
Cohen 1994	50	-0.48(0.94)	91	-0.62(0.94)		45.7	0.14[-0.18,0.46]
Dewey 1999	59	-1.09(0.89)	60	-1.17(0.76)		54.3	0.08[-0.22,0.38]
Total(95%CI)	109		151			100.0	0.11[-0.11,0.33]
Test for heterogeneity chi-square=0.07 df=1 p=0.79							
Test for overall effect z=0.96 p=0.3							

-1 -.5 0 .5 1
Favours MBF   Favours EBF

Comparison: 01 Exclusive vs mixed breastfeeding 4-6 months, developing countries, controlled trials
Outcome: 07 Weight-for-length z-score at 6 months

Study	EBF n	mean(sd)	MBF n	mean(sd)	WMD (95%CI Fixed)	Weight %	WMD (95%CI Fixed)
Cohen 1994	50	0.60(0.74)	91	0.49(0.95)		60.0	0.11[-0.17,0.39]
Dewey 1999	59	0.12(0.93)	60	0.06(1.00)		40.0	0.06[-0.29,0.41]
Total(95%CI)	109		151			100.0	0.09[-0.13,0.31]
Test for heterogeneity chi-square=0.05 df=1 p=0.83							
Test for overall effect z=0.80 p=0.4							

-1 -.5 0 .5 1
Favours MBF   Favours EBF

Comparison: 01 Exclusive vs mixed breastfeeding 4-6 months, developing countries, controlled trials
Outcome: 08 Weight-for-age z-score <-2 at 6 months

Study	EBF n/N	MBF n/N	RR (95%CI Fixed)	Weight %	RR (95%CI Fixed)
Cohen 1994	2 / 50	0 / 91		8.2	9.02[0.44,184.28]
Dewey 1999	6 / 59	4 / 60		91.8	1.53[0.45,5.13]
Total(95%CI)	8 / 109	4 / 151		100.0	2.14[0.74,6.24]
Test for heterogeneity chi-square=1.17 df=1 p=0.28					
Test for overall effect z=1.40 p=0.16					

.001 .02 1 50 1000
Favours EBF   Favours MBF

Comparison: 01 Exclusive vs mixed breastfeeding 4-6 months, developing countries, controlled trials
Outcome: 09 Length-for-age z-score <-2 at 6 months

Study	EBF n/N	MBF n/N	RR (95%CI Fixed)	Weight %	RR (95%CI Fixed)
Cohen 1994	4 / 50	6 / 91		38.0	1.21[0.36,4.10]
Dewey 1999	8 / 59	7 / 60		62.0	1.16[0.45,3.00]
Total(95%CI)	12 / 109	13 / 151		100.0	1.18[0.56,2.50]
Test for heterogeneity chi-square=0.00 df=1 p=0.96					
Test for overall effect z=0.44 p=0.7					

.1 .2 1 5 10
Favours EBF   Favours MBF

Comparison: 01 Exclusive vs mixed breastfeeding 4-6 months, developing countries, controlled trials
Outcome: 10 Weight-for-length z-score < -2 at 6 months

Study	EBF n/N	MBF n/N	RR (95%CI Fixed)	Weight %	RR (95%CI Fixed)
Cohen 1994	0 / 50	1 / 91		68.3	0.60[0.02,14.49]
Dewey 1999	1 / 59	0 / 60		31.7	3.05[0.13,73.40]
Total(95%CI)	1 / 109	1 / 151		100.0	1.38[0.17,10.98]

Test for heterogeneity chi-square=0.50 df=1 p=0.48
Test for overall effect z=0.30 p=0.8

.001 .02 1 50 1000
Favours EBF   Favours MBF

Comparison: 01 Exclusive vs mixed breastfeeding 4-6 months, developing countries, controlled trials
Outcome: 11 Receipt of Fe supplements 6-9 months

Study	EBF n/N	MBF n/N	RR (95%CI Fixed)	Weight %	RR (95%CI Fixed)
Cohen 1994	33 / 50	49 / 89		100.0	1.20[0.91,1.58]
Total(95%CI)	33 / 50	49 / 89		100.0	1.20[0.91,1.58]

Test for heterogeneity chi-square=0.0 df=0
Test for overall effect z=1.30 p=0.19

.5 .7 1 1.5 2
Favours EBF   Favours MBF

Comparison: 01 Exclusive vs mixed breastfeeding 4-6 months, developing countries, controlled trials
Outcome: 12 Hemoglobin concentration (g/L) at 6 months

Study	EBF n	EBF mean(sd)	MBF n	MBF mean(sd)	WMD (95%CI Fixed)	Weight %	WMD (95%CI Fixed)
Cohen 1994	50	104.00(10.00)	89	109.00(10.00)		100.0	-5.00[-8.46,-1.54]
Total(95%CI)	50		89			100.0	-5.00[-8.46,-1.54]

Test for heterogeneity chi-square=0.0 df=0
Test for overall effect z=2.83 p=0.005

-10 -5 0 5 10
Favours MBF   Favours EBF

Comparison: 01 Exclusive vs mixed breastfeeding 4-6 months, developing countries, controlled trials
Outcome: 13 Hemoglobin concentration <110 g/L at 6 months

Study	EBF n/N	MBF n/N	RR (95%CI Fixed)	Weight %	RR (95%CI Fixed)
Cohen 1994	33 / 50	49 / 89		100.0	1.20[0.91,1.58]
Total(95%CI)	33 / 50	49 / 89		100.0	1.20[0.91,1.58]

Test for heterogeneity chi-square=0.0 df=0
Test for overall effect z=1.30 p=0.19

.5 .7 1 1.5 2
Favours EBF   Favours MBF

Comparison: 01 Exclusive vs mixed breastfeeding 4-6 months, developing countries, controlled trials
Outcome: 14 Hemoglobin concentration <103 g/L at 6 months

Study	EBF n/N	MBF n/N	RR (95%CI Fixed)	Weight %	RR (95%CI Fixed)
Cohen 1994	16 / 50	22 / 89		100.0	1.29[0.75,2.23]
Total(95%CI)	16 / 50	22 / 89		100.0	1.29[0.75,2.23]

Test for heterogeneity chi-square=0.0 df=0
Test for overall effect z=0.93 p=0.4

.2 .5 1 2 5
Favours EBF   Favours MBF

Comparison: 01 Exclusive vs mixed breastfeeding 4-6 months, developing countries, controlled trials
Outcome: 15 Hematocrit (%) at 6 months

Study	EBF n	mean(sd)	MBF n	mean(sd)	WMD (95%CI Fixed)	Weight %	WMD (95%CI Fixed)
Cohen 1994	50	33.50(2.80)	89	34.70(2.60)		100.0	-1.20[-2.15,-0.25]
Total(95%CI)	50		89			100.0	-1.20[-2.15,-0.25]

Test for heterogeneity chi-square=0.0 df=0
Test for overall effect z=2.49 p=0.01

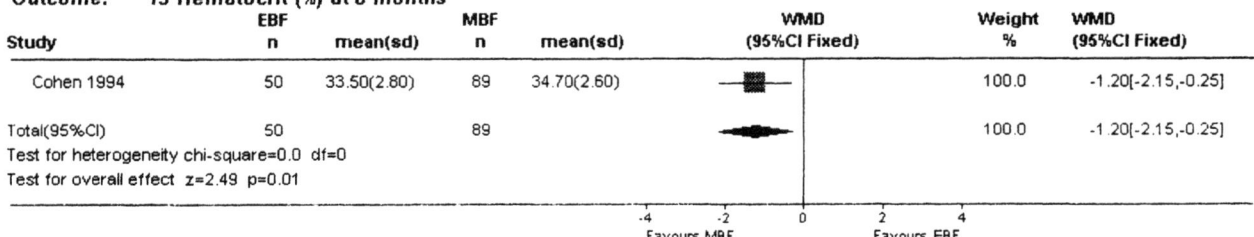

Comparison: 01 Exclusive vs mixed breastfeeding 4-6 months, developing countries, controlled trials
Outcome: 16 Hematocrit <33% at 6 months

Study	EBF n/N	MBF n/N	RR (95%CI Fixed)	Weight %	RR (95%CI Fixed)
Cohen 1994	16 / 50	19 / 89		100.0	1.50[0.85,2.64]
Total(95%CI)	16 / 50	19 / 89		100.0	1.50[0.85,2.64]

Test for heterogeneity chi-square=0.0 df=0
Test for overall effect z=1.40 p=0.16

Comparison: 01 Exclusive vs mixed breastfeeding 4-6 months, developing countries, controlled trials
Outcome: 17 Plasma ferritin concentration (mcg/L) at 6 months

Study	EBF n	mean(sd)	MBF n	mean(sd)	WMD (95%CI Fixed)	Weight %	WMD (95%CI Fixed)
Cohen 1994	49	48.40(44.20)	86	67.30(64.50)		100.0	-18.90[-37.31,-0.49]
Total(95%CI)	49		86			100.0	-18.90[-37.31,-0.49]

Test for heterogeneity chi-square=0.0 df=0
Test for overall effect z=2.01 p=0.04

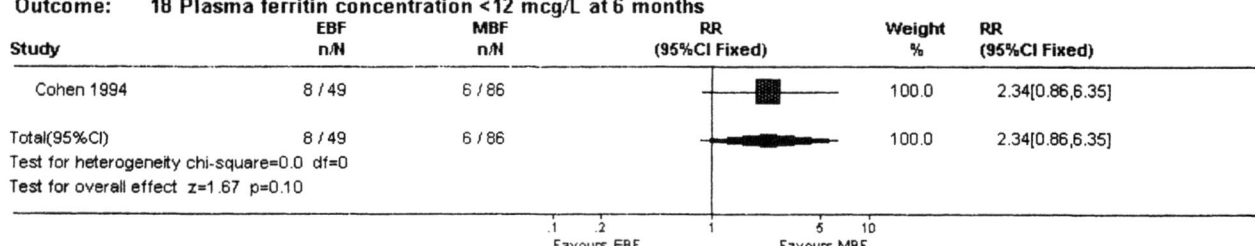

Comparison: 01 Exclusive vs mixed breastfeeding 4-6 months, developing countries, controlled trials
Outcome: 18 Plasma ferritin concentration <12 mcg/L at 6 months

Study	EBF n/N	MBF n/N	RR (95%CI Fixed)	Weight %	RR (95%CI Fixed)
Cohen 1994	8 / 49	6 / 86		100.0	2.34[0.86,6.35]
Total(95%CI)	8 / 49	6 / 86		100.0	2.34[0.86,6.35]

Test for heterogeneity chi-square=0.0 df=0
Test for overall effect z=1.67 p=0.10

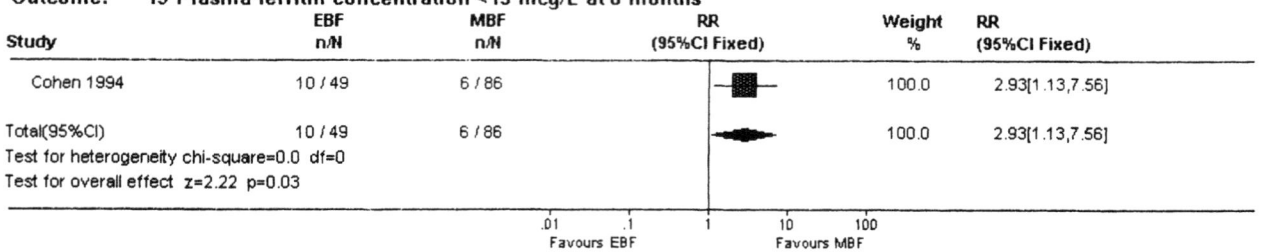

Comparison: 01 Exclusive vs mixed breastfeeding 4-6 months, developing countries, controlled trials
Outcome: 19 Plasma ferritin concentration <15 mcg/L at 6 months

Study	EBF n/N	MBF n/N	RR (95%CI Fixed)	Weight %	RR (95%CI Fixed)
Cohen 1994	10 / 49	6 / 86		100.0	2.93[1.13,7.56]
Total(95%CI)	10 / 49	6 / 86		100.0	2.93[1.13,7.56]

Test for heterogeneity chi-square=0.0 df=0
Test for overall effect z=2.22 p=0.03

Comparison: 01 Exclusive vs mixed breastfeeding 4-6 months, developing countries, controlled trials
Outcome: 20 Plasma zinc concentration <70 mcg/dL at 6 months

Study	EBF n/N	MBF n/N	RR (95%CI Fixed)	Weight %	RR (95%CI Fixed)
Dewey 1999	15 / 53	18 / 48		100.0	0.75[0.43,1.33]
Total(95%CI)	15 / 53	18 / 48		100.0	0.75[0.43,1.33]

Test for heterogeneity chi-square=0.0 df=0
Test for overall effect z=-0.98 p=0.3

Favours EBF / Favours MBF

Comparison: 01 Exclusive vs mixed breastfeeding 4-6 months, developing countries, controlled trials
Outcome: 21 % of days with fever 4-6 months

Study	EBF n	mean(sd)	MBF n	mean(sd)	WMD (95%CI Fixed)	Weight %	WMD (95%CI Fixed)
Cohen 1994	50	5.65(5.42)	91	5.61(5.63)		66.9	0.04[-1.86,1.94]
Dewey 1999	59	8.00(7.20)	60	7.30(7.80)		33.1	0.70[-2.00,3.40]
Total(95%CI)	109		151			100.0	0.26[-1.29,1.81]

Test for heterogeneity chi-square=0.15 df=1 p=0.69
Test for overall effect z=0.33 p=0.7

Favours EBF / Favours MBF

Comparison: 01 Exclusive vs mixed breastfeeding 4-6 months, developing countries, controlled trials
Outcome: 22 % of days with cough 4-6 months

Study	EBF n	mean(sd)	MBF n	mean(sd)	WMD (95%CI Fixed)	Weight %	WMD (95%CI Fixed)
Cohen 1994	50	28.54(20.39)	91	21.10(17.74)		56.2	7.44[0.71,14.17]
Dewey 1999	59	26.10(20.30)	60	29.20(22.10)		43.8	-3.10[-10.72,4.52]
Total(95%CI)	109		151			100.0	2.83[-2.22,7.87]

Test for heterogeneity chi-square=4.13 df=1 p=0.042
Test for overall effect z=1.10 p=0.3

Favours EBF / Favours MBF

Comparison: 01 Exclusive vs mixed breastfeeding 4-6 months, developing countries, controlled trials
Outcome: 23 % of days with nasal congestion 4-6 months

Study	EBF n	mean(sd)	MBF n	mean(sd)	WMD (95%CI Fixed)	Weight %	WMD (95%CI Fixed)
Cohen 1994	50	22.25(18.12)	91	19.49(15.25)		58.4	2.76[-3.16,8.68]
Dewey 1999	59	15.40(15.00)	60	19.00(23.20)		41.6	-3.60[-10.61,3.41]
Total(95%CI)	109		151			100.0	0.11[-4.41,4.63]

Test for heterogeneity chi-square=1.85 df=1 p=0.17
Test for overall effect z=0.05 p=1

Favours EBF / Favours MBF

Comparison: 01 Exclusive vs mixed breastfeeding 4-6 months, developing countries, controlled trials
Outcome: 24 % of days with nasal discharge 4-6 months

Study	EBF n	mean(sd)	MBF n	mean(sd)	WMD (95%CI Fixed)	Weight %	WMD (95%CI Fixed)
Cohen 1994	50	8.69(10.26)	91	6.63(8.94)		71.3	2.06[-1.33,5.45]
Dewey 1999	59	12.00(12.20)	60	16.20(17.10)		28.7	-4.20[-9.53,1.13]
Total(95%CI)	109		151			100.0	0.26[-2.60,3.12]

Test for heterogeneity chi-square=3.78 df=1 p=0.052
Test for overall effect z=0.18 p=0.9

Favours EBF / Favours MBF

Comparison: 01 Exclusive vs mixed breastfeeding 4-6 months, developing countries, controlled trials
Outcome: 25 % of days with hoarseness 4-6 months

Study	EBF n	mean(sd)	MBF n	mean(sd)	WMD (95%CI Fixed)	Weight %	WMD (95%CI Fixed)
Cohen 1994	50	1.44(2.73)	91	1.66(4.10)		74.5	-0.22[-1.35,0.91]
Dewey 1999	59	2.50(4.30)	60	2.60(6.30)		25.5	-0.10[-2.04,1.84]
Total(95%CI)	109		151			100.0	-0.19[-1.17,0.79]

Test for heterogeneity chi-square=0.01 df=1 p=0.92
Test for overall effect z=0.38 p=0.7

-4 -2 0 2 4
Favours EBF   Favours MBF

Comparison: 01 Exclusive vs mixed breastfeeding 4-6 months, developing countries, controlled trials
Outcome: 26 % of days with diarrhea 4-6 months

Study	EBF n	mean(sd)	MBF n	mean(sd)	WMD (95%CI Fixed)	Weight %	WMD (95%CI Fixed)
Cohen 1994	50	4.15(5.69)	91	3.76(4.72)		65.7	0.39[-1.46,2.24]
Dewey 1999	59	5.40(8.50)	60	2.80(5.40)		34.3	2.60[0.04,5.16]
Total(95%CI)	109		151			100.0	1.15[-0.35,2.65]

Test for heterogeneity chi-square=1.88 df=1 p=0.17
Test for overall effect z=1.50 p=0.13

-10 -5 0 5 10
Favours EBF   Favours MBF

Comparison: 01 Exclusive vs mixed breastfeeding 4-6 months, developing countries, controlled trials
Outcome: 27 % of days with fever 6-12 months

Study	EBF n	mean(sd)	MBF n	mean(sd)	WMD (95%CI Fixed)	Weight %	WMD (95%CI Fixed)
Cohen 1994	49	9.48(9.49)	91	9.44(8.49)		57.5	0.04[-3.14,3.22]
Dewey 1999	58	8.21(8.94)	60	9.18(11.43)		42.5	-0.97[-4.67,2.73]
Total(95%CI)	107		151			100.0	-0.39[-2.80,2.02]

Test for heterogeneity chi-square=0.16 df=1 p=0.68
Test for overall effect z=0.32 p=0.8

-10 -5 0 5 10
Favours EBF   Favours MBF

Comparison: 01 Exclusive vs mixed breastfeeding 4-6 months, developing countries, controlled trials
Outcome: 28 % of days with nasal congestion 6-12 months

Study	EBF n	mean(sd)	MBF n	mean(sd)	WMD (95%CI Fixed)	Weight %	WMD (95%CI Fixed)
Cohen 1994	49	9.01(11.57)	91	6.75(10.31)		69.9	2.26[-1.61,6.13]
Dewey 1999	58	15.62(19.64)	60	10.53(12.02)		30.1	5.09[-0.81,10.99]
Total(95%CI)	107		151			100.0	3.11[-0.12,6.35]

Test for heterogeneity chi-square=0.62 df=1 p=0.43
Test for overall effect z=1.88 p=0.06

-10 -5 0 5 10
Favours EBF   Favours MBF

Comparison: 01 Exclusive vs mixed breastfeeding 4-6 months, developing countries, controlled trials
Outcome: 29 % of days with diarrhea 6-12 months

Study	EBF n	mean(sd)	MBF n	mean(sd)	WMD (95%CI Fixed)	Weight %	WMD (95%CI Fixed)
Cohen 1994	49	3.15(5.77)	91	3.70(6.68)		56.8	-0.55[-2.67,1.57]
Dewey 1999	58	3.72(6.02)	60	4.71(7.40)		43.2	-0.99[-3.42,1.44]
Total(95%CI)	107		151			100.0	-0.74[-2.34,0.86]

Test for heterogeneity chi-square=0.07 df=1 p=0.79
Test for overall effect z=0.91 p=0.4

-10 -5 0 5 10
Favours EBF   Favours MBF

Comparison: 01 Exclusive vs mixed breastfeeding 4-6 months, developing countries, controlled trials
Outcome: 30 Age first crawled (mo)

Study	EBF n	mean(sd)	MBF n	mean(sd)	WMD (95%CI Fixed)	Weight %	WMD (95%CI Fixed)
Cohen 1994	47	6.30(1.80)	89	7.25(1.56)		56.6	-0.95[-1.56,-0.34]
Dewey 1999	54	6.80(1.70)	50	7.40(1.90)		43.4	-0.60[-1.29,0.09]
Total(95%CI)	101		139			100.0	-0.80[-1.26,-0.34]

Test for heterogeneity chi-square=0.55 df=1 p=0.46
Test for overall effect z=3.42 p=0.0006

-4 -2 0 2 4
Favours EBF   Favours MBF

Comparison: 01 Exclusive vs mixed breastfeeding 4-6 months, developing countries, controlled trials
Outcome: 31 Age first sat from lying position (mo)

Study	EBF n	mean(sd)	MBF n	mean(sd)	WMD (95%CI Fixed)	Weight %	WMD (95%CI Fixed)
Cohen 1994	46	7.00(1.50)	89	6.90(1.15)		60.9	0.10[-0.39,0.59]
Dewey 1999	53	7.40(1.60)	50	8.00(1.60)		39.1	-0.60[-1.22,0.02]
Total(95%CI)	99		139			100.0	-0.17[-0.56,0.21]

Test for heterogeneity chi-square=3.00 df=1 p=0.083
Test for overall effect z=0.88 p=0.4

-4 -2 0 2 4
Favours EBF   Favours MBF

Comparison: 01 Exclusive vs mixed breastfeeding 4-6 months, developing countries, controlled trials
Outcome: 32 Did not walk by 12 months

Study	EBF n/N	MBF n/N	RR (95%CI Fixed)	Weight %	RR (95%CI Fixed)
Cohen 1994	19/47	53/87		50.6	0.66[0.45,0.98]
Dewey 1999	41/50	36/49		49.4	1.12[0.90,1.38]
Total(95%CI)	60/97	89/136		100.0	0.89[0.72,1.09]

Test for heterogeneity chi-square=6.65 df=1 p=0.0099
Test for overall effect z=-1.14 p=0.3

.1 .2 1 5 10
Favours EBF   Favours MBF

Comparison: 01 Exclusive vs mixed breastfeeding 4-6 months, developing countries, controlled trials
Outcome: 33 Maternal postpartum weight loss 4-6 months (kg)

Study	EBF n	mean(sd)	MBF n	mean(sd)	WMD (95%CI Fixed)	Weight %	WMD (95%CI Fixed)
Cohen 1994	50	0.70(1.50)	91	0.10(1.70)		54.4	0.60[0.06,1.14]
Dewey 1999	59	0.30(1.60)	60	0.10(1.70)		45.6	0.20[-0.39,0.79]
Total(95%CI)	109		151			100.0	0.42[0.02,0.82]

Test for heterogeneity chi-square=0.95 df=1 p=0.33
Test for overall effect z=2.04 p=0.04

-4 -2 0 2 4
Favours MBF   Favours EBF

Comparison: 01 Exclusive vs mixed breastfeeding 4-6 months, developing countries, controlled trials
Outcome: 34 Maternal resumption of menses 6 months postpartum

Study	EBF n/N	MBF n/N	RR (95%CI Fixed)	Weight %	RR (95%CI Fixed)
Cohen 1994	8/40	16/66		48.1	0.82[0.39,1.75]
Dewey 1999	5/45	12/38		51.9	0.35[0.14,0.91]
Total(95%CI)	13/85	28/104		100.0	0.58[0.33,1.03]

Test for heterogeneity chi-square=1.91 df=1 p=0.17
Test for overall effect z=-1.85 p=0.06

.1 .2 1 5 10
Favours EBF   Favours MBF

ANNEX 2

Comparison 02: Exclusive vs mixed breastfeeding 3-7 months, developing countries, observational studies

Comparison: 02 Exclusive vs mixed breastfeeding 3-7 months, developing countries, observational studies
Outcome: 01 Monthly weight gain 4-6 months (g/mo)

Study	EBF n	mean(sd)	MBF n	mean(sd)	WMD (95%CI Fixed)	Weight %	WMD (95%CI Fixed)
Adair 1993	370	336.00(157.00)	834	350.00(167.00)		86.7	-14.00[-33.61,5.61]
Brown 1991	15	402.00(198.00)	21	359.00(168.00)		2.2	43.00[-80.30,166.30]
Simondon 1997	154	324.80(250.00)	216	288.90(286.00)		11.1	35.90[-19.00,90.80]
Total(95%CI)	539		1071			100.0	-7.23[-25.49,11.03]

Test for heterogeneity chi-square=3.47 df=2 p=0.18
Test for overall effect z=0.78 p=0.4

-100 -50 0 50 100
Favours MBF   Favours EBF

Comparison: 02 Exclusive vs mixed breastfeeding 3-7 months, developing countries, observational studies
Outcome: 02 Monthly weight gain 6-9 months (g/mo)

Study	EBF n	mean(sd)	MBF n	mean(sd)	WMD (95%CI Fixed)	Weight %	WMD (95%CI Fixed)
Simondon 1997	129	190.00(210.00)	190	196.00(223.00)		100.0	-6.00[-54.15,42.15]
Total(95%CI)	129		190			100.0	-6.00[-54.15,42.15]

Test for heterogeneity chi-square=0.0 df=0
Test for overall effect z=0.24 p=0.8

-100 -50 0 50 100
Favours MBF   Favours EBF

Comparison: 02 Exclusive vs mixed breastfeeding 3-7 months, developing countries, observational studies
Outcome: 03 Monthly length gain 4-6 months (cm/mo)

Study	EBF n	mean(sd)	MBF n	mean(sd)	WMD (95%CI Fixed)	Weight %	WMD (95%CI Fixed)
Adair 1993	370	1.60(0.80)	834	1.60(0.75)		58.4	0.00[-0.10,0.10]
Brown 1991	15	1.63(0.27)	21	1.57(0.44)		10.0	0.06[-0.17,0.29]
Simondon 1997	154	1.55(0.66)	216	1.43(0.59)		31.6	0.12[-0.01,0.25]
Total(95%CI)	539		1071			100.0	0.04[-0.03,0.12]

Test for heterogeneity chi-square=2.12 df=2 p=0.35
Test for overall effect z=1.17 p=0.2

-.5 -.25 0 .25 .5
Favours MBF   Favours EBF

Comparison: 02 Exclusive vs mixed breastfeeding 3-7 months, developing countries, observational studies
Outcome: 04 Monthly length gain 6-9 months (cm/mo)

Study	EBF n	mean(sd)	MBF n	mean(sd)	WMD (95%CI Fixed)	Weight %	WMD (95%CI Fixed)
Simondon 1997	129	1.28(0.42)	190	1.24(0.44)		100.0	0.04[-0.06,0.14]
Total(95%CI)	129		190			100.0	0.04[-0.06,0.14]

Test for heterogeneity chi-square=0.0 df=0
Test for overall effect z=0.82 p=0.4

-.5 -.25 0 .25 .5
Favours MBF   Favours EBF

Comparison: 02 Exclusive vs mixed breastfeeding 3-7 months, developing countries, observational studies
Outcome: 05 Weight-for-age z-score at 6-7 months

Study	EBF n	mean(sd)	MBF n	mean(sd)	WMD (95%CI Fixed)	Weight %	WMD (95%CI Fixed)
Simondon 1997	154	-0.71(1.02)	216	-0.84(1.09)		100.0	0.13[-0.09,0.35]
Total(95%CI)	154		216			100.0	0.13[-0.09,0.35]

Test for heterogeneity chi-square=0.0 df=0
Test for overall effect z=1.17 p=0.2

-1 -.5 0 .5 1
Favours MBF   Favours EBF

Comparison: 02 Exclusive vs mixed breastfeeding 3-7 months, developing countries, observational studies
Outcome: 06 Weight-for-age z-score at 9-10 month

Study	EBF n	mean(sd)	MBF n	mean(sd)	WMD (95%CI Fixed)	Weight %	WMD (95%CI Fixed)
Simondon 1997	129	-1.37(1.13)	190	-1.46(0.97)		100.0	0.09[-0.15,0.33]
Total(95%CI)	129		190			100.0	0.09[-0.15,0.33]

Test for heterogeneity chi-square=0.00 df=0 p=1
Test for overall effect z=0.74 p=0.5

-1 -.5 0 .5 1
Favours MBF   Favours EBF

Comparison: 02 Exclusive vs mixed breastfeeding 3-7 months, developing countries, observational studies
Outcome: 07 Length-for-age z-score at 6-7 months

Study	EBF n	mean(sd)	MBF n	mean(sd)	WMD (95%CI Fixed)	Weight %	WMD (95%CI Fixed)
Simondon 1997	154	-0.76(0.89)	216	-0.80(0.86)		100.0	0.04[-0.14,0.22]
Total(95%CI)	154		216			100.0	0.04[-0.14,0.22]

Test for heterogeneity chi-square=0.0 df=0
Test for overall effect z=0.43 p=0.7

-1 -.5 0 .5 1
Favours MBF   Favours EBF

Comparison: 02 Exclusive vs mixed breastfeeding 3-7 months, developing countries, observational studies
Outcome: 08 Length-for-age z-score at 9-10 months

Study	EBF n	mean(sd)	MBF n	mean(sd)	WMD (95%CI Fixed)	Weight %	WMD (95%CI Fixed)
Simondon 1997	129	-0.90(0.91)	190	-1.01(0.91)		100.0	0.11[-0.09,0.31]
Total(95%CI)	129		190			100.0	0.11[-0.09,0.31]

Test for heterogeneity chi-square=0.0 df=0
Test for overall effect z=1.06 p=0.3

-1 -.5 0 .5 1
Favours MBF   Favours EBF

Comparison: 02 Exclusive vs mixed breastfeeding 3-7 months, developing countries, observational studies
Outcome: 09 Weight-for-length z-score at 6-7 months

Study	EBF n	mean(sd)	MBF n	mean(sd)	WMD (95%CI Fixed)	Weight %	WMD (95%CI Fixed)
Simondon 1997	154	-0.18(0.96)	216	-0.29(0.98)		100.0	0.11[-0.09,0.31]
Total(95%CI)	154		216			100.0	0.11[-0.09,0.31]

Test for heterogeneity chi-square=0.0 df=0
Test for overall effect z=1.08 p=0.3

-1 -.5 0 .5 1
Favours MBF   Favours EBF

Comparison: 02 Exclusive vs mixed breastfeeding 3-7 months, developing countries, observational studies
Outcome: 10 Weight-for-length z-score at 9-10 months

Study	EBF n	mean(sd)	MBF n	mean(sd)	WMD (95%CI Fixed)	Weight %	WMD (95%CI Fixed)
Simondon 1997	129	-0.83(1.04)	190	-0.84(0.84)		100.0	0.01[-0.21,0.23]
Total(95%CI)	129		190			100.0	0.01[-0.21,0.23]

Test for heterogeneity chi-square=0.0 df=0
Test for overall effect z=0.09 p=0.9

Favours MBF / Favours EBF

Comparison: 02 Exclusive vs mixed breastfeeding 3-7 months, developing countries, observational studies
Outcome: 11 Weight-for-age z-score < -2 at 6-7 months

Study	EBF n/N	MBF n/N	RR (95%CI Fixed)	Weight %	RR (95%CI Fixed)
Simondon 1997	19 / 154	29 / 216		100.0	0.92[0.54,1.58]
Total(95%CI)	19 / 154	29 / 216		100.0	0.92[0.54,1.58]

Test for heterogeneity chi-square=0.0 df=0
Test for overall effect z=-0.31 p=0.8

Favours EBF / Favours MBF

Comparison: 02 Exclusive vs mixed breastfeeding 3-7 months, developing countries, observational studies
Outcome: 12 Weight-for-age z-score < -2 at 9-10 months

Study	EBF n/N	MBF n/N	RR (95%CI Fixed)	Weight %	RR (95%CI Fixed)
Simondon 1997	33 / 129	52 / 190		100.0	0.93[0.64,1.36]
Total(95%CI)	33 / 129	52 / 190		100.0	0.93[0.64,1.36]

Test for heterogeneity chi-square=0.0 df=0
Test for overall effect z=-0.35 p=0.7

Favours EBF / Favours MBF

Comparison: 02 Exclusive vs mixed breastfeeding 3-7 months, developing countries, observational studies
Outcome: 13 Length-for-age z-score < -2 at 6-7 months

Study	EBF n/N	MBF n/N	RR (95%CI Fixed)	Weight %	RR (95%CI Fixed)
Simondon 1997	12 / 154	14 / 216		100.0	1.20[0.57,2.53]
Total(95%CI)	12 / 154	14 / 216		100.0	1.20[0.57,2.53]

Test for heterogeneity chi-square=0.0 df=0
Test for overall effect z=0.49 p=0.6

Favours EBF / Favours MBF

Comparison: 02 Exclusive vs mixed breastfeeding 3-7 months, developing countries, observational studies
Outcome: 14 Length-for-age z-score < -2 at 9-10 months

Study	EBF n/N	MBF n/N	RR (95%CI Fixed)	Weight %	RR (95%CI Fixed)
Simondon 1997	14 / 129	17 / 190		100.0	1.21[0.62,2.37]
Total(95%CI)	14 / 129	17 / 190		100.0	1.21[0.62,2.37]

Test for heterogeneity chi-square=0.0 df=0
Test for overall effect z=0.56 p=0.6

Favours EBF / Favours MBF

Comparison: 02 Exclusive vs mixed breastfeeding 3-7 months, developing countries, observational studies
Outcome: 15 Weight-for-length z-score < -2 at 6-7 months

Study	EBF n/N	MBF n/N	RR (95%CI Fixed)	Weight %	RR (95%CI Fixed)
Simondon 1997	3 / 154	10 / 216		100.0	0.42[0.12,1.50]
Total(95%CI)	3 / 154	10 / 216		100.0	0.42[0.12,1.50]

Test for heterogeneity chi-square=0.0 df=0
Test for overall effect z=-1.33 p=0.18

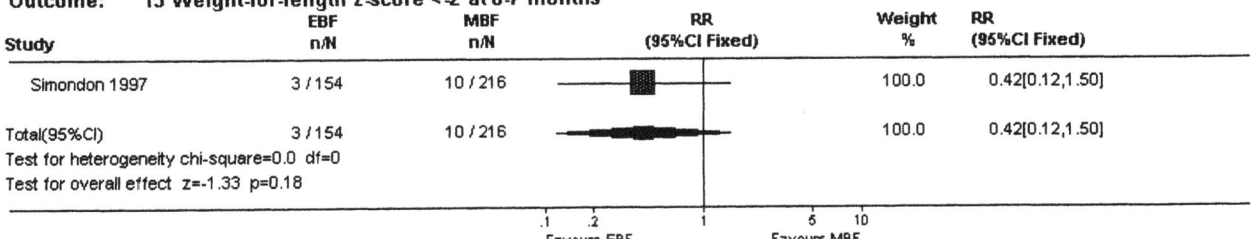

Comparison: 02 Exclusive vs mixed breastfeeding 3-7 months, developing countries, observational studies
Outcome: 16 Weight-for-length z-score < -2 at 9-10 months

Study	EBF n/N	MBF n/N	RR (95%CI Fixed)	Weight %	RR (95%CI Fixed)
Simondon 1997	10 / 129	18 / 190		100.0	0.82[0.39,1.72]
Total(95%CI)	10 / 129	18 / 190		100.0	0.82[0.39,1.72]

Test for heterogeneity chi-square=0.0 df=0
Test for overall effect z=-0.53 p=0.6

Comparison: 02 Exclusive vs mixed breastfeeding 3-7 months, developing countries, observational studies
Outcome: 17 Mid-upper arm circumference at 6-7 months (cm)

Study	EBF n	mean(sd)	MBF n	mean(sd)	WMD (95%CI Fixed)	Weight %	WMD (95%CI Fixed)
Simondon 1997	154	13.30(1.10)	216	13.10(1.20)		100.0	0.20[-0.04,0.44]
Total(95%CI)	154		216			100.0	0.20[-0.04,0.44]

Test for heterogeneity chi-square=0.00 df=0 p=1
Test for overall effect z=1.66 p=0.10

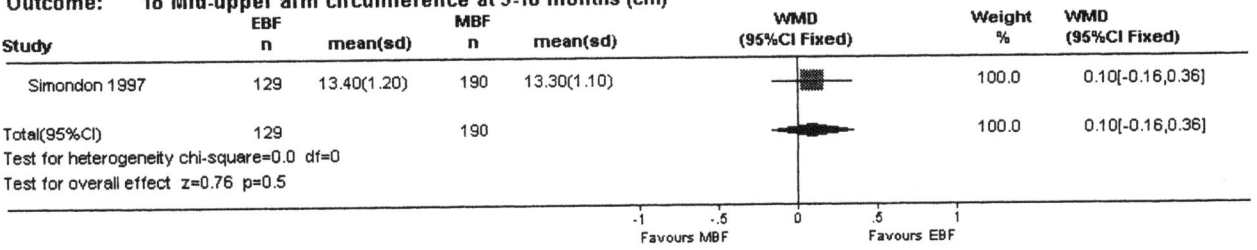

Comparison: 02 Exclusive vs mixed breastfeeding 3-7 months, developing countries, observational studies
Outcome: 18 Mid-upper arm circumference at 9-10 months (cm)

Study	EBF n	mean(sd)	MBF n	mean(sd)	WMD (95%CI Fixed)	Weight %	WMD (95%CI Fixed)
Simondon 1997	129	13.40(1.20)	190	13.30(1.10)		100.0	0.10[-0.16,0.36]
Total(95%CI)	129		190			100.0	0.10[-0.16,0.36]

Test for heterogeneity chi-square=0.0 df=0
Test for overall effect z=0.76 p=0.5

ANNEX 3

Comparison 03: Exclusive vs mixed breastfeeding 3-7 months, developed countries, observational studies

Comparison: 03 Exclusive vs mixed breastfeeding 3-7 months, developed countries, observational studies
Outcome: 01 Monthly weight gain 3-8 months (g/mo)

Study	EBF n	EBF mean(sd)	MBF n	MBF mean(sd)	Weight %	WMD (95%CI Fixed)
Akeson 1996	10	498.00(118.00)	9	438.00(127.00)	1.0	60.00[-50.61,170.61]
Kramer 2000	619	612.20(180.00)	2836	641.00(186.00)	48.9	-28.80[-44.55,-13.05]
WHO 1994	200	463.00(142.00)	158	470.00(159.00)	12.1	-7.00[-38.65,24.65]
WHO 1997	179	418.75(100.39)	377	413.80(100.39)	38.0	4.95[-12.91,22.81]
Total(95%CI)	1008		3380		100.0	-12.45[-23.47,-1.44]

Test for heterogeneity chi-square=9.55 df=3 p=0.023
Test for overall effect z=2.22 p=0.03

Comparison: 03 Exclusive vs mixed breastfeeding 3-7 months, developed countries, observational studies
Outcome: 02 Monthly weight gain 6-9 months (g/mo)

Study	EBF n	EBF mean(sd)	MBF n	MBF mean(sd)	Weight %	WMD (95%CI Fixed)
Heinig 1993	17	322.00(103.00)	33	259.00(124.00)	5.1	63.00[-1.71,127.71]
Kramer 2000	611	449.70(171.00)	2771	455.50(177.00)	94.9	-5.80[-20.88,9.28]
Total(95%CI)	628		2804		100.0	-2.26[-16.94,12.42]

Test for heterogeneity chi-square=4.12 df=1 p=0.042
Test for overall effect z=0.30 p=0.8

Comparison: 03 Exclusive vs mixed breastfeeding 3-7 months, developed countries, observational studies
Outcome: 03 Monthly weight gain 8-12 months (g/mo)

Study	EBF n	EBF mean(sd)	MBF n	MBF mean(sd)	Weight %	WMD (95%CI Fixed)
Akeson 1996	3	282.00(88.00)	5	288.00(93.00)	1.3	-6.00[-134.69,122.69]
Heinig 1993	15	241.00(104.00)	31	240.00(126.00)	4.7	1.00[-67.83,69.83]
Kramer 2000	609	353.90(176.00)	2787	355.80(172.00)	94.0	-1.90[-17.27,13.47]
Total(95%CI)	627		2823		100.0	-1.82[-16.72,13.08]

Test for heterogeneity chi-square=0.01 df=2 p=0.99
Test for overall effect z=0.24 p=0.8

Comparison: 03 Exclusive vs mixed breastfeeding 3-7 months, developed countries, observational studies
Outcome: 04 Monthly length gain 3-8 months (cm/mo)

Study	EBF n	EBF mean(sd)	MBF n	MBF mean(sd)	Weight %	WMD (95%CI Fixed)
Akeson 1996	10	1.80(0.24)	9	1.68(0.30)	2.0	0.12[-0.13,0.37]
Kramer 2000	618	1.93(0.64)	2836	2.04(0.70)	38.4	-0.11[-0.17,-0.05]
WHO 1994	200	1.72(0.43)	156	1.76(0.48)	13.3	-0.04[-0.14,0.06]
WHO 1997	179	1.87(0.29)	377	1.85(0.29)	46.3	0.02[-0.03,0.07]
Total(95%CI)	1007		3378		100.0	-0.04[-0.07,0.00]

Test for heterogeneity chi-square=12.63 df=3 p=0.0055
Test for overall effect z=2.00 p=0.05

Comparison: 03 Exclusive vs mixed breastfeeding 3-7 months, developed countries, observational studies
Outcome: 05 Monthly length gain 6-9 months (cm/mo)

Study	EBF n	mean(sd)	MBF n	mean(sd)	WMD (95%CI Fixed)	Weight %	WMD (95%CI Fixed)
Heinig 1993	17	1.40(0.40)	33	1.30(0.30)		6.5	0.10[-0.12,0.32]
Kramer 2000	610	1.49(0.65)	2770	1.54(0.65)		93.5	-0.05[-0.11,0.01]
Total(95%CI)	627		2803			100.0	-0.04[-0.10,0.01]

Test for heterogeneity chi-square=1.73 df=1 p=0.19
Test for overall effect z=1.43 p=0.15

-.5 -.25 0 .25 .5
Favours MBF   Favours EBF

Comparison: 03 Exclusive vs mixed breastfeeding 3-7 months, developed countries, observational studies
Outcome: 06 Monthly length gain 8-12 months (cm/mo)

Study	EBF n	mean(sd)	MBF n	mean(sd)	WMD (95%CI Fixed)	Weight %	WMD (95%CI Fixed)
Akeson 1996	3	1.32(0.27)	5	1.32(0.27)		2.1	0.00[-0.39,0.39]
Heinig 1993	15	1.40(0.30)	31	1.30(0.30)		9.0	0.10[-0.08,0.28]
Kramer 2000	608	1.43(0.68)	2786	1.34(0.63)		88.9	0.09[0.03,0.15]
Total(95%CI)	626		2822			100.0	0.09[0.03,0.14]

Test for heterogeneity chi-square=0.22 df=2 p=0.9
Test for overall effect z=3.14 p=0.002

-.5 -.25 0 .25 .5
Favours MBF   Favours EBF

Comparison: 03 Exclusive vs mixed breastfeeding 3-7 months, developed countries, observational studies
Outcome: 07 Weight-for-age z-score at 6 months

Study	EBF n	mean(sd)	MBF n	mean(sd)	WMD (95%CI Fixed)	Weight %	WMD (95%CI Fixed)
Kramer 2000	619	0.54(0.84)	2836	0.63(0.83)		100.0	-0.09[-0.16,-0.02]
Total(95%CI)	619		2836			100.0	-0.09[-0.16,-0.02]

Test for heterogeneity chi-square=0.0 df=0
Test for overall effect z=2.42 p=0.02

-.5 -.25 0 .25 .5
Favours MBF   Favours EBF

Comparison: 03 Exclusive vs mixed breastfeeding 3-7 months, developed countries, observational studies
Outcome: 08 Weight-for-age z-score at 9 months

Study	EBF n	mean(sd)	MBF n	mean(sd)	WMD (95%CI Fixed)	Weight %	WMD (95%CI Fixed)
Kramer 2000	611	0.49(0.88)	2789	0.59(0.86)		100.0	-0.10[-0.18,-0.02]
Total(95%CI)	611		2789			100.0	-0.10[-0.18,-0.02]

Test for heterogeneity chi-square=0.0 df=0
Test for overall effect z=2.55 p=0.01

-.5 -.25 0 .25 .5
Favours MBF   Favours EBF

Comparison: 03 Exclusive vs mixed breastfeeding 3-7 months, developed countries, observational studies
Outcome: 09 Weight-for-age z-score at 12 months

Study	EBF n	mean(sd)	MBF n	mean(sd)	WMD (95%CI Fixed)	Weight %	WMD (95%CI Fixed)
Kramer 2000	616	0.54(0.94)	2842	0.63(0.86)		100.0	-0.09[-0.17,-0.01]
Total(95%CI)	616		2842			100.0	-0.09[-0.17,-0.01]

Test for heterogeneity chi-square=0.0 df=0
Test for overall effect z=2.19 p=0.03

-.5 -.25 0 .25 .5
Favours MBF   Favours EBF

Comparison: 03 Exclusive vs mixed breastfeeding 3-7 months, developed countries, observational studies
Outcome: 10 Length-for-age z-score at 6 months

Study	EBF n	mean(sd)	MBF n	mean(sd)	WMD (95%CI Fixed)	Weight %	WMD (95%CI Fixed)
Kramer 2000	618	-0.05(0.95)	2836	0.07(0.94)		100.0	-0.12[-0.20,-0.04]
Total(95%CI)	618		2836			100.0	-0.12[-0.20,-0.04]

Test for heterogeneity chi-square=0.0 df=0
Test for overall effect z=2.85 p=0.004

-.5 -.25 0 .25 .5
Favours MBF   Favours EBF

Comparison: 03 Exclusive vs mixed breastfeeding 3-7 months, developed countries, observational studies
Outcome: 11 Length-for-age z-score at 9 months

Study	EBF n	mean(sd)	MBF n	mean(sd)	WMD (95%CI Fixed)	Weight %	WMD (95%CI Fixed)
Kramer 2000	610	-0.05(0.97)	2788	0.09(0.96)		100.0	-0.14[-0.22,-0.06]
Total(95%CI)	610		2788			100.0	-0.14[-0.22,-0.06]

Test for heterogeneity chi-square=0.0 df=0
Test for overall effect z=3.23 p=0.001

-.5 -.25 0 .25 .5
Favours MBF   Favours EBF

Comparison: 03 Exclusive vs mixed breastfeeding 3-7 months, developed countries, observational studies
Outcome: 12 Length-for-age z-score at 12 months

Study	EBF n	mean(sd)	MBF n	mean(sd)	WMD (95%CI Fixed)	Weight %	WMD (95%CI Fixed)
Kramer 2000	616	0.13(0.90)	2842	0.15(0.91)		100.0	-0.02[-0.10,0.06]
Total(95%CI)	616		2842			100.0	-0.02[-0.10,0.06]

Test for heterogeneity chi-square=0.0 df=0
Test for overall effect z=0.50 p=0.6

-.5 -.25 0 .25 .5
Favours MBF   Favours EBF

Comparison: 03 Exclusive vs mixed breastfeeding 3-7 months, developed countries, observational studies
Outcome: 13 Weight-for-length z-score at 6 months

Study	EBF n	mean(sd)	MBF n	mean(sd)	WMD (95%CI Fixed)	Weight %	WMD (95%CI Fixed)
Kramer 2000	618	0.65(0.97)	2836	0.63(1.01)		100.0	0.02[-0.07,0.11]
Total(95%CI)	618		2836			100.0	0.02[-0.07,0.11]

Test for heterogeneity chi-square=0.00 df=0 p=1
Test for overall effect z=0.46 p=0.6

-.5 -.25 0 .25 .5
Favours MBF   Favours EBF

Comparison: 03 Exclusive vs mixed breastfeeding 3-7 months, developed countries, observational studies
Outcome: 14 Weight-for-length z-score at 9 months

Study	EBF n	mean(sd)	MBF n	mean(sd)	WMD (95%CI Fixed)	Weight %	WMD (95%CI Fixed)
Kramer 2000	610	0.75(0.98)	2788	0.72(0.99)		100.0	0.03[-0.06,0.12]
Total(95%CI)	610		2788			100.0	0.03[-0.06,0.12]

Test for heterogeneity chi-square=0.00 df=0 p=1
Test for overall effect z=0.68 p=0.5

-.5 -.25 0 .25 .5
Favours MBF   Favours EBF

ANNEX 3. COMPARISON 03

Comparison: 03 Exclusive vs mixed breastfeeding 3-7 months, developed countries, observational studies
Outcome: 15 Weight-for-length z-score at 12 months

Study	EBF n	mean(sd)	MBF n	mean(sd)	WMD (95%CI Fixed)	Weight %	WMD (95%CI Fixed)
Kramer 2000	616	0.71(0.99)	2842	0.79(0.95)		100.0	-0.08[-0.17,0.01]
Total(95%CI)	616		2842			100.0	-0.08[-0.17,0.01]

Test for heterogeneity chi-square=0.0 df=0
Test for overall effect z=1.83 p=0.07

Favours MBF / Favours EBF

Comparison: 03 Exclusive vs mixed breastfeeding 3-7 months, developed countries, observational studies
Outcome: 16 Weight-for-age z-score <-2 at 6 months

Study	EBF n/N	MBF n/N	RR (95%CI Fixed)	Weight %	RR (95%CI Fixed)
Kramer 2000	0 / 620	2 / 2841		100.0	0.92[0.04,19.04]
Total(95%CI)	0 / 620	2 / 2841		100.0	0.92[0.04,19.04]

Test for heterogeneity chi-square=0.0 df=0
Test for overall effect z=-0.06 p=1

Favours EBF / Favours MBF

Comparison: 03 Exclusive vs mixed breastfeeding 3-7 months, developed countries, observational studies
Outcome: 17 Weight-for-age z-score <-2 at 9 months

Study	EBF n/N	MBF n/N	RR (95%CI Fixed)	Weight %	RR (95%CI Fixed)
Kramer 2000	1 / 612	3 / 2796		100.0	1.52[0.16,14.62]
Total(95%CI)	1 / 612	3 / 2796		100.0	1.52[0.16,14.62]

Test for heterogeneity chi-square=0.0 df=0
Test for overall effect z=0.36 p=0.7

Favours EBF / Favours MBF

Comparison: 03 Exclusive vs mixed breastfeeding 3-7 months, developed countries, observational studies
Outcome: 18 Weight-for-age z-score <-2 at 12 months

Study	EBF n/N	MBF n/N	RR (95%CI Fixed)	Weight %	RR (95%CI Fixed)
Kramer 2000	1 / 617	4 / 2849		100.0	1.15[0.13,10.31]
Total(95%CI)	1 / 617	4 / 2849		100.0	1.15[0.13,10.31]

Test for heterogeneity chi-square=0.0 df=0
Test for overall effect z=0.13 p=0.9

Favours EBF / Favours MBF

Comparison: 03 Exclusive vs mixed breastfeeding 3-7 months, developed countries, observational studies
Outcome: 19 Length-for-age z-score <-2 at 6 months

Study	EBF n/N	MBF n/N	RR (95%CI Fixed)	Weight %	RR (95%CI Fixed)
Kramer 2000	14 / 619	42 / 2841		100.0	1.53[0.84,2.78]
Total(95%CI)	14 / 619	42 / 2841		100.0	1.53[0.84,2.78]

Test for heterogeneity chi-square=0.0 df=0
Test for overall effect z=1.39 p=0.16

Favours EBF / Favours MBF

Comparison: 03 Exclusive vs mixed breastfeeding 3-7 months, developed countries, observational studies
Outcome: 20 Length-for-age z-score < -2 at 9 months

Study	EBF n/N	MBF n/N	RR (95%CI Fixed)	Weight %	RR (95%CI Fixed)
Kramer 2000	14 / 611	44 / 2795		100.0	1.46[0.80,2.64]
Total(95%CI)	14 / 611	44 / 2795		100.0	1.46[0.80,2.64]
Test for heterogeneity chi-square=0.0 df=0					
Test for overall effect z=1.24 p=0.2					

.1 .2   1   5 10
Favours EBF   Favours MBF

Comparison: 03 Exclusive vs mixed breastfeeding 3-7 months, developed countries, observational studies
Outcome: 21 Length-for-age z-score < -2 at 12 months

Study	EBF n/N	MBF n/N	RR (95%CI Fixed)	Weight %	RR (95%CI Fixed)
Kramer 2000	4 / 617	28 / 2849		100.0	0.66[0.23,1.87]
Total(95%CI)	4 / 617	28 / 2849		100.0	0.66[0.23,1.87]
Test for heterogeneity chi-square=0.0 df=0					
Test for overall effect z=-0.78 p=0.4					

.1 .2   1   5 10
Favours EBF   Favours MBF

Comparison: 03 Exclusive vs mixed breastfeeding 3-7 months, developed countries, observational studies
Outcome: 22 Weight-for-length z-score < -2 at 6 months

Study	EBF n/N	MBF n/N	RR (95%CI Fixed)	Weight %	RR (95%CI Fixed)
Kramer 2000	0 / 619	7 / 2841		100.0	0.31[0.02,5.34]
Total(95%CI)	0 / 619	7 / 2841		100.0	0.31[0.02,5.34]
Test for heterogeneity chi-square=0.0 df=0					
Test for overall effect z=-0.81 p=0.4					

.001 .02   1   50 1000
Favours EBF   Favours MBF

Comparison: 03 Exclusive vs mixed breastfeeding 3-7 months, developed countries, observational studies
Outcome: 23 Weight-for-length z-score < -2 at 9 months

Study	EBF n/N	MBF n/N	RR (95%CI Fixed)	Weight %	RR (95%CI Fixed)
Kramer 2000	2 / 611	8 / 2795		100.0	1.14[0.24,5.37]
Total(95%CI)	2 / 611	8 / 2795		100.0	1.14[0.24,5.37]
Test for heterogeneity chi-square=0.0 df=0					
Test for overall effect z=0.17 p=0.9					

.01 .1   1   10 100
Favours EBF   Favours MBF

Comparison: 03 Exclusive vs mixed breastfeeding 3-7 months, developed countries, observational studies
Outcome: 24 Weight-for-length z-score < -2 at 12 months

Study	EBF n/N	MBF n/N	RR (95%CI Fixed)	Weight %	RR (95%CI Fixed)
Kramer 2000	1 / 617	4 / 2849		100.0	1.15[0.13,10.31]
Total(95%CI)	1 / 617	4 / 2849		100.0	1.15[0.13,10.31]
Test for heterogeneity chi-square=0.0 df=0					
Test for overall effect z=0.13 p=0.9					

.01 .1   1   10 100
Favours EBF   Favours MBF

Comparison: 03 Exclusive vs mixed breastfeeding 3-7 months, developed countries, observational studies
Outcome: 25 Head circumference at 6 months (cm)

Study	EBF n	mean(sd)	MBF n	mean(sd)	WMD (95%CI Fixed)	Weight %	WMD (95%CI Fixed)
Kramer 2000	615	43.34(1.53)	2825	43.44(1.46)		100.0	-0.10[-0.23,0.03]
Total(95%CI)	615		2825			100.0	-0.10[-0.23,0.03]

Test for heterogeneity chi-square=0.00 df=0 p=1
Test for overall effect z=1.48 p=0.14

-.5 -.25 0 .25 .5
Favours MBF   Favours EBF

Comparison: 03 Exclusive vs mixed breastfeeding 3-7 months, developed countries, observational studies
Outcome: 26 Head circumference at 9 months (cm)

Study	EBF n	mean(sd)	MBF n	mean(sd)	WMD (95%CI Fixed)	Weight %	WMD (95%CI Fixed)
Kramer 2000	609	45.52(1.46)	2780	45.45(1.43)		100.0	0.07[-0.06,0.20]
Total(95%CI)	609		2780			100.0	0.07[-0.06,0.20]

Test for heterogeneity chi-square=0.0 df=0
Test for overall effect z=1.08 p=0.3

-.5 -.25 0 .25 .5
Favours MBF   Favours EBF

Comparison: 03 Exclusive vs mixed breastfeeding 3-7 months, developed countries, observational studies
Outcome: 27 Head circumference at 12 months (cm)

Study	EBF n	mean(sd)	MBF n	mean(sd)	WMD (95%CI Fixed)	Weight %	WMD (95%CI Fixed)
Kramer 2000	614	47.25(1.50)	2836	47.06(1.49)		100.0	0.19[0.06,0.32]
Total(95%CI)	614		2836			100.0	0.19[0.06,0.32]

Test for heterogeneity chi-square=0.0 df=0
Test for overall effect z=2.85 p=0.004

-.5 -.25 0 .25 .5
Favours MBF   Favours EBF

Comparison: 03 Exclusive vs mixed breastfeeding 3-7 months, developed countries, observational studies
Outcome: 28 Sleeping time at 9 months (min/day)

Study	EBF n	mean(sd)	MBF n	mean(sd)	WMD (95%CI Fixed)	Weight %	WMD (95%CI Fixed)
Heinig 1993	17	729.00(66.00)	33	728.00(61.00)		100.0	1.00[-36.65,38.65]
Total(95%CI)	17		33			100.0	1.00[-36.65,38.65]

Test for heterogeneity chi-square=0.0 df=0
Test for overall effect z=0.05 p=1

-100 -50 0 50 100
Favours MBF   Favours EBF

Comparison: 03 Exclusive vs mixed breastfeeding 3-7 months, developed countries, observational studies
Outcome: 29 Total essential amino acid concentration (umol/L) at 6 months

Study	EBF n	mean(sd)	MBF n	mean(sd)	WMD (95%CI Fixed)	Weight %	WMD (95%CI Fixed)
Akeson 1996	26	1045.00(150.00)	18	1023.00(125.00)		100.0	22.00[-59.60,103.60]
Total(95%CI)	26		18			100.0	22.00[-59.60,103.60]

Test for heterogeneity chi-square=0.0 df=0
Test for overall effect z=0.53 p=0.6

-1000 -500 0 500 1000
Favours MBF   Favours EBF

Comparison: 03 Exclusive vs mixed breastfeeding 3-7 months, developed countries, observational studies
Outcome: 30 Total amino acid concentration (umol/L) at 6 months

Study	EBF n	mean(sd)	MBF n	mean(sd)	WMD (95%CI Fixed)	Weight %	WMD (95%CI Fixed)
Akeson 1996	26	2974.00(331.00)	18	2901.00(309.00)		100.0	73.00[-118.22,264.22]
Total(95%CI)	26		18			100.0	73.00[-118.22,264.22]
Test for heterogeneity chi-square=0.0 df=0							
Test for overall effect z=0.75 p=0.5							

-1000 -500 0 500 1000
Favours MBF   Favours EBF

Comparison: 03 Exclusive vs mixed breastfeeding 3-7 months, developed countries, observational studies
Outcome: 31 Atopic eczema in first 12 months

Study	EBF n/N	MBF n/N	RR (95%CI Fixed)	Weight %	RR (95%CI Fixed)
Kajosaari 1983	10 / 70	23 / 65		46.2	0.40[0.21,0.78]
Kramer 2000	17 / 621	78 / 2862		53.8	1.00[0.60,1.69]
Total(95%CI)	27 / 691	101 / 2927		100.0	0.73[0.49,1.08]
Test for heterogeneity chi-square=4.54 df=1 p=0.033					
Test for overall effect z=-1.57 p=0.12					

.1 .2 1 5 10
Favours EBF   Favours MBF

Comparison: 03 Exclusive vs mixed breastfeeding 3-7 months, developed countries, observational studies
Outcome: 32 Food allergy at 1 year (by history)

Study	EBF n/N	MBF n/N	RR (95%CI Fixed)	Weight %	RR (95%CI Fixed)
Kajosaari 1983	5 / 70	24 / 65		100.0	0.19[0.08,0.48]
Total(95%CI)	5 / 70	24 / 65		100.0	0.19[0.08,0.48]
Test for heterogeneity chi-square=0.0 df=0					
Test for overall effect z=-3.57 p=0.0004					

.01 .1 1 10 100
Favours EBF   Favours MBF

Comparison: 03 Exclusive vs mixed breastfeeding 3-7 months, developed countries, observational studies
Outcome: 33 Food allergy at 1 year (by double challenge)

Study	EBF n/N	MBF n/N	RR (95%CI Fixed)	Weight %	RR (95%CI Fixed)
Kajosaari 1983	5 / 70	6 / 65		100.0	0.77[0.25,2.41]
Total(95%CI)	5 / 70	6 / 65		100.0	0.77[0.25,2.41]
Test for heterogeneity chi-square=0.0 df=0					
Test for overall effect z=-0.44 p=0.7					

.1 .2 1 5 10
Favours EBF   Favours MBF

Comparison: 03 Exclusive vs mixed breastfeeding 3-7 months, developed countries, observational studies
Outcome: 34 Two or more episodes of wheezing in first 12 months

Study	EBF n/N	MBF n/N	RR (95%CI Fixed)	Weight %	RR (95%CI Fixed)
Kramer 2000	2 / 621	6 / 2862		6.5	1.54[0.31,7.59]
Oddy 1999	22 / 246	32 / 264		93.5	0.74[0.44,1.23]
Total(95%CI)	24 / 867	38 / 3126		100.0	0.79[0.49,1.28]
Test for heterogeneity chi-square=0.73 df=1 p=0.39					
Test for overall effect z=-0.95 p=0.3					

.1 .2 1 5 10
Favours EBF   Favours MBF

ANNEX 3. COMPARISON 03

Comparison: 03 Exclusive vs mixed breastfeeding 3-7 months, developed countries, observational studies
Outcome: 35 Any atopy at 5 years

Study	EBF n/N	MBF n/N	RR (95%CI Fixed)	Weight %	RR (95%CI Fixed)
Kajosaari 1983	14 / 51	25 / 62		100.0	0.68[0.40,1.17]
Total(95%CI)	14 / 51	25 / 62		100.0	0.68[0.40,1.17]

Test for heterogeneity chi-square=0.0 df=0
Test for overall effect z=-1.40 p=0.16

.2 .5 1 2 5
Favours EBF   Favours MBF

Comparison: 03 Exclusive vs mixed breastfeeding 3-7 months, developed countries, observational studies
Outcome: 36 Atopic eczema at 5 years

Study	EBF n/N	MBF n/N	RR (95%CI Fixed)	Weight %	RR (95%CI Fixed)
Kajosaari 1983	12 / 51	15 / 62		100.0	0.97[0.50,1.89]
Total(95%CI)	12 / 51	15 / 62		100.0	0.97[0.50,1.89]

Test for heterogeneity chi-square=0.0 df=0
Test for overall effect z=-0.08 p=0.9

.2 .5 1 2 5
Favours EBF   Favours MBF

Comparison: 03 Exclusive vs mixed breastfeeding 3-7 months, developed countries, observational studies
Outcome: 37 Pollen allergy at 5 years

Study	EBF n/N	MBF n/N	RR (95%CI Fixed)	Weight %	RR (95%CI Fixed)
Kajosaari 1983	10 / 51	23 / 62		100.0	0.53[0.28,1.01]
Total(95%CI)	10 / 51	23 / 62		100.0	0.53[0.28,1.01]

Test for heterogeneity chi-square=0.0 df=0
Test for overall effect z=-1.94 p=0.05

.2 .5 1 2 5
Favours EBF   Favours MBF

Comparison: 03 Exclusive vs mixed breastfeeding 3-7 months, developed countries, observational studies
Outcome: 38 Asthma at 5-6 years

Study	EBF n/N	MBF n/N	RR (95%CI Fixed)	Weight %	RR (95%CI Fixed)
Kajosaari 1983	4 / 51	9 / 62		18.9	0.54[0.18,1.65]
Oddy 1999	33 / 207	37 / 232		81.1	1.00[0.65,1.54]
Total(95%CI)	37 / 258	46 / 294		100.0	0.91[0.61,1.36]

Test for heterogeneity chi-square=1.02 df=1 p=0.31
Test for overall effect z=-0.45 p=0.7

.1 .2 1 5 10
Favours EBF   Favours MBF

Comparison: 03 Exclusive vs mixed breastfeeding 3-7 months, developed countries, observational studies
Outcome: 39 Food allergy at 5 years (by history)

Study	EBF n/N	MBF n/N	RR (95%CI Fixed)	Weight %	RR (95%CI Fixed)
Kajosaari 1983	2 / 51	4 / 62		100.0	0.61[0.12,3.19]
Total(95%CI)	2 / 51	4 / 62		100.0	0.61[0.12,3.19]

Test for heterogeneity chi-square=0.0 df=0
Test for overall effect z=-0.59 p=0.6

.01 .1 1 10 100
Favours EBF   Favours MBF

Comparison: 03 Exclusive vs mixed breastfeeding 3-7 months, developed countries, observational studies
Outcome: 40 Allergy to animal dander at 5 years

Study	EBF n/N	MBF n/N	RR (95%CI Fixed)	Weight %	RR (95%CI Fixed)
Kajosaari 1983	4 / 51	6 / 62		100.0	0.81[0.24,2.72]
Total(95%CI)	4 / 51	6 / 62		100.0	0.81[0.24,2.72]

Test for heterogeneity chi-square=0.0 df=0
Test for overall effect z=-0.34 p=0.7

.01 .1 1 10 100
Favours EBF   Favours MBF

Comparison: 03 Exclusive vs mixed breastfeeding 3-7 months, developed countries, observational studies
Outcome: 41 Positive skin prick test at 6 years

Study	EBF n/N	MBF n/N	RR (95%CI Fixed)	Weight %	RR (95%CI Fixed)
Oddy 1999	53 / 160	57 / 171		100.0	0.99[0.73,1.35]
Total(95%CI)	53 / 160	57 / 171		100.0	0.99[0.73,1.35]

Test for heterogeneity chi-square=0.0 df=0
Test for overall effect z=-0.04 p=1

.5 .7 1 1.5 2
Favours EBF   Favours MBF

Comparison: 03 Exclusive vs mixed breastfeeding 3-7 months, developed countries, observational studies
Outcome: 42 Hemoglobin concentration (g/L) at 12 months

Study	EBF n	mean(sd)	MBF n	mean(sd)	WMD (95%CI Fixed)	Weight %	WMD (95%CI Fixed)
Pisacane 1995	9	117.00(4.00)	21	109.00(7.00)		100.0	8.00[4.03,11.97]
Total(95%CI)	9		21			100.0	8.00[4.03,11.97]

Test for heterogeneity chi-square=0.0 df=0
Test for overall effect z=3.95 p=0.00008

-100 -50 0 50 100
Favours MBF   Favours EBF

Comparison: 03 Exclusive vs mixed breastfeeding 3-7 months, developed countries, observational studies
Outcome: 43 Hemoglobin concentration <110 g/L at 12 months

Study	EBF n/N	MBF n/N	RR (95%CI Fixed)	Weight %	RR (95%CI Fixed)
Pisacane 1995	0 / 9	9 / 21		100.0	0.12[0.01,1.80]
Total(95%CI)	0 / 9	9 / 21		100.0	0.12[0.01,1.80]

Test for heterogeneity chi-square=0.0 df=0
Test for overall effect z=-1.54 p=0.12

.001 .02 1 50 1000
Favours EBF   Favours MBF

Comparison: 03 Exclusive vs mixed breastfeeding 3-7 months, developed countries, observational studies
Outcome: 44 Serum ferritin concentration (mcg/L) at 12 months

Study	EBF n	mean(sd)	MBF n	mean(sd)	WMD (95%CI Fixed)	Weight %	WMD (95%CI Fixed)
Pisacane 1995	9	17.00(15.00)	21	12.30(11.70)		100.0	4.70[-6.30,15.70]
Total(95%CI)	9		21			100.0	4.70[-6.30,15.70]

Test for heterogeneity chi-square=0.0 df=0
Test for overall effect z=0.84 p=0.4

-100 -50 0 50 100
Favours MBF   Favours EBF

Comparison: 03 Exclusive vs mixed breastfeeding 3-7 months, developed countries, observational studies
Outcome: 45 Serum ferritin concetration <10 mcg/L at 12 months

Study	EBF n/N	MBF n/N	RR (95%CI Fixed)	Weight %	RR (95%CI Fixed)
Pisacane 1995	2 / 9	11 / 21		100.0	0.42[0.12,1.54]
Total(95%CI)	2 / 9	11 / 21		100.0	0.42[0.12,1.54]
Test for heterogeneity chi-square=0.0 df=0					
Test for overall effect z=-1.30 p=0.19					

.01 .1 1 10 100
Favours EBF   Favours MBF

Comparison: 03 Exclusive vs mixed breastfeeding 3-7 months, developed countries, observational studies
Outcome: 46 Death in first 12 months

Study	EBF n/N	MBF n/N	RR (95%CI Fixed)	Weight %	RR (95%CI Fixed)
Kramer 2000	1 / 621	2 / 2862		100.0	2.30[0.21,25.37]
Total(95%CI)	1 / 621	2 / 2862		100.0	2.30[0.21,25.37]
Test for heterogeneity chi-square=0.0 df=0					
Test for overall effect z=0.68 p=0.5					

.01 .1 1 10 100
Favours EBF   Favours MBF

Comparison: 03 Exclusive vs mixed breastfeeding 3-7 months, developed countries, observational studies
Outcome: 47 One or more episodes of gastrointestinal infection in first 12 months

Study	EBF n/N	MBF n/N	RR (95%CI Fixed)	Weight %	RR (95%CI Fixed)
Kramer 2000	31 / 621	213 / 2862		100.0	0.67[0.46,0.97]
Total(95%CI)	31 / 621	213 / 2862		100.0	0.67[0.46,0.97]
Test for heterogeneity chi-square=0.0 df=0					
Test for overall effect z=-2.13 p=0.03					

.1 .2 1 5 10
Favours EBF   Favours MBF

Comparison: 03 Exclusive vs mixed breastfeeding 3-7 months, developed countries, observational studies
Outcome: 48 Hospitalization for gastrointestinal infection in first 12 months

Study	EBF n/N	MBF n/N	RR (95%CI Fixed)	Weight %	RR (95%CI Fixed)
Kramer 2000	11 / 621	64 / 2862		100.0	0.79[0.42,1.49]
Total(95%CI)	11 / 621	64 / 2862		100.0	0.79[0.42,1.49]
Test for heterogeneity chi-square=0.0 df=0					
Test for overall effect z=-0.72 p=0.5					

.1 .2 1 5 10
Favours EBF   Favours MBF

Comparison: 03 Exclusive vs mixed breastfeeding 3-7 months, developed countries, observational studies
Outcome: 49 One or more episodes of upper respiratory tract infection in first 12 months

Study	EBF n/N	MBF n/N	RR (95%CI Fixed)	Weight %	RR (95%CI Fixed)
Oddy 1999	179 / 246	179 / 264		100.0	1.07[0.96,1.20]
Total(95%CI)	179 / 246	179 / 264		100.0	1.07[0.96,1.20]
Test for heterogeneity chi-square=0.0 df=0					
Test for overall effect z=1.23 p=0.2					

.5 .7 1 1.5 2
Favours EBF   Favours MBF

Comparison: 03 Exclusive vs mixed breastfeeding 3-7 months, developed countries, observational studies
Outcome: 50 Two or more episodes of upper respiratory tract infection in first 12 months

Study	EBF n/N	MBF n/N	RR (95%CI Fixed)	Weight %	RR (95%CI Fixed)
Kramer 2000	175 / 621	887 / 2862		71.3	0.91 [0.79, 1.04]
Oddy 1999	114 / 246	132 / 264		28.7	0.93 [0.77, 1.11]
Total(95%CI)	289 / 867	1019 / 3126		100.0	0.91 [0.82, 1.02]

Test for heterogeneity chi-square=0.03 df=1 p=0.87
Test for overall effect z=-1.59 p=0.11

.5   .7   1   1.5   2
Favours EBF   Favours MBF

Comparison: 03 Exclusive vs mixed breastfeeding 3-7 months, developed countries, observational studies
Outcome: 51 Four or more episodes of upper respiratory tract infection in first 12 months

Study	EBF n/N	MBF n/N	RR (95%CI Fixed)	Weight %	RR (95%CI Fixed)
Oddy 1999	29 / 246	38 / 264		100.0	0.82 [0.52, 1.29]
Total(95%CI)	29 / 246	38 / 264		100.0	0.82 [0.52, 1.29]

Test for heterogeneity chi-square=0.0 df=0
Test for overall effect z=-0.87 p=0.4

.5   .7   1   1.5   2
Favours EBF   Favours MBF

Comparison: 03 Exclusive vs mixed breastfeeding 3-7 months, developed countries, observational studies
Outcome: 52 One or more episodes of lower respiratory tract infection in first 12 months

Study	EBF n/N	MBF n/N	RR (95%CI Fixed)	Weight %	RR (95%CI Fixed)
Oddy 1999	107 / 264	93 / 246		100.0	1.07 [0.86, 1.33]
Total(95%CI)	107 / 264	93 / 246		100.0	1.07 [0.86, 1.33]

Test for heterogeneity chi-square=0.0 df=0
Test for overall effect z=0.63 p=0.5

.5   .7   1   1.5   2
Favours EBF   Favours MBF

Comparison: 03 Exclusive vs mixed breastfeeding 3-7 months, developed countries, observational studies
Outcome: 53 Two or more episodes of respiratory tract infection (upper or lower) in first 12 months

Study	EBF n/N	MBF n/N	RR (95%CI Fixed)	Weight %	RR (95%CI Fixed)
Kramer 2000	190 / 621	969 / 2862		100.0	0.90 [0.79, 1.03]
Total(95%CI)	190 / 621	969 / 2862		100.0	0.90 [0.79, 1.03]

Test for heterogeneity chi-square=0.0 df=0
Test for overall effect z=-1.54 p=0.12

.5   .7   1   1.5   2
Favours EBF   Favours MBF

Comparison: 03 Exclusive vs mixed breastfeeding 3-7 months, developed countries, observational studies
Outcome: 54 Hospitalization for respiratory tract infection in first 12 months

Study	EBF n/N	MBF n/N	RR (95%CI Fixed)	Weight %	RR (95%CI Fixed)
Kramer 2000	69 / 621	411 / 2862		89.4	0.77 [0.61, 0.98]
Oddy 1999	9 / 246	18 / 264		10.6	0.54 [0.25, 1.17]
Total(95%CI)	78 / 867	429 / 3126		100.0	0.75 [0.60, 0.94]

Test for heterogeneity chi-square=0.77 df=1 p=0.38
Test for overall effect z=-2.48 p=0.01

.1   .2   1   5   10
Favours EBF   Favours MBF

Comparison: 03 Exclusive vs mixed breastfeeding 3-7 months, developed countries, observational studies
Outcome: 55 Number of episodes of otitis media in first 12 months

Study	EBF n	mean(sd)	MBF n	mean(sd)	WMD (95%CI Fixed)	Weight %	WMD (95%CI Fixed)
Duncan 1993	138	1.48(1.95)	141	1.52(1.85)		100.0	-0.04[-0.49,0.41]
Total(95%CI)	138		141			100.0	-0.04[-0.49,0.41]

Test for heterogeneity chi-square=0.0 df=0
Test for overall effect z=0.18 p=0.9

Favours EBF / Favours MBF

Comparison: 03 Exclusive vs mixed breastfeeding 3-7 months, developed countries, observational studies
Outcome: 56 One or more episodes of otitis media in first 12 months

Study	EBF n/N	MBF n/N	RR (95%CI Fixed)	Weight %	RR (95%CI Fixed)
Duncan 1993	75/138	60/141		53.1	1.28[1.00,1.63]
Kramer 2000	41/621	147/2862		46.9	1.29[0.92,1.80]
Total(95%CI)	116/759	207/3003		100.0	1.28[1.04,1.57]

Test for heterogeneity chi-square=0.00 df=1 p=0.98
Test for overall effect z=2.38 p=0.02

Favours EBF / Favours MBF

Comparison: 03 Exclusive vs mixed breastfeeding 3-7 months, developed countries, observational studies
Outcome: 57 Frequent otitis media in first 12 months

Study	EBF n/N	MBF n/N	RR (95%CI Fixed)	Weight %	RR (95%CI Fixed)
Duncan 1993	15/138	19/141		100.0	0.81[0.43,1.52]
Total(95%CI)	15/138	19/141		100.0	0.81[0.43,1.52]

Test for heterogeneity chi-square=0.0 df=0
Test for overall effect z=-0.66 p=0.5

Favours EBF / Favours MBF

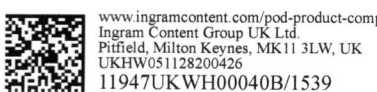

www.ingramcontent.com/pod-product-compliance
Ingram Content Group UK Ltd.
Pitfield, Milton Keynes, MK11 3LW, UK
UKHW051128200426
11947UKWH00040B/1539

9 789241 595643